SHADOW WORK

First published in 2024 by Wellfleet Press,
an imprint of The Quarto Group,
142 West 36th Street, 4th Floor,
New York, NY 10018, USA
T (212) 779-4972
www.Quarto.com

Contains content previously published in 2022 as *A Guide to Shadow Work* by Wellfleet Press,
an imprint of The Quarto Group, 142 West 36th Street, 4th Floor, New York, NY 10018, USA

Wellfleet titles are also available at discount for retail, wholesale, promotional, and bulk purchase. For details, contact the Special Sales Manager by email at specialsales@quarto.com or by mail at The Quarto Group, Attn: Special Sales Manager, 100 Cummings Center Suite 265D, Beverly, MA 01915 USA.

10 9 8 7 6 5 4 3 2 1

ISBN: 978-0-7603-8880-8

Library of Congress Cataloging-in-Publication Data

Names: Kirby, Stephanie, author.
Title: Shadow work : your personal guide / Stephanie Kirby.
Description: New York, NY : Wellfleet Press, [2024] | Series: In focus |
   Includes bibliographical references and index. | Summary: "In Focus
   Shadow Work is the essential modern guide to shadow work, the healing
   path to understanding and embracing the dark side of your personality"—
   Provided by publisher.
Identifiers: LCCN 2023049308 | ISBN 9780760388808 (hardcover)
Subjects: LCSH: Self-realization. | Personality. | Jungian psychology.
Classification: LCC BF637.S4 K5533 2024 | DDC 158.1—dc23/eng/20231206
LC record available at https://lccn.loc.gov/2023049308

Publisher: Rage Kindelsperger
Editorial Director: Erin Canning
Creative Director: Laura Drew
Managing Editor: Cara Donaldson
Editor: Sara Bonacum
Cover and Interior Design: Ashley Prine/Tandem Books

Printed in China

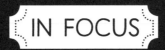

SHADOW WORK

Your Personal Guide

STEPHANIE KIRBY

wellfleet
press

CONTENTS

INTRODUCTION

The shadow is your so-called "dark side"; however, you will soon understand why that is an inaccurate description. The shadow is actually your disowned and repressed self—it is not inherently dark or negative. It is an archetypal figure in mythology, literature, and religion. Encounters with the shadow are often described by metaphors such as dancing with the devil, battling inner demons, slaying the dragon, or the dark night of the soul. I like to think of the shadow as my dark sidekick rather than my dark side because this slight differentiation reminds me that the shadow is in fact working with me rather than against me, although it doesn't always feel like it.

The Psychology of the Shadow

Carl Jung is a psychologist credited with discovering the shadow in Western psychology. However, the concept of the shadow has been around for centuries. Before Jung, the shadow was primarily known through fables, myths, religious texts, and archetypal figures. Jung's shadow concept evolved from Sigmund Freud's analysis of the split between the light and dark sides of the human psyche. Jung's understanding of the shadow evolved over many years—as early as 1912, he used the term "shadow side of the psyche." According to Jung, the less you are aware of what lies within your shadow, the denser and darker it is. He believed that until you become aware of what exists within the unconscious it is impossible to become the steward of your own mind.

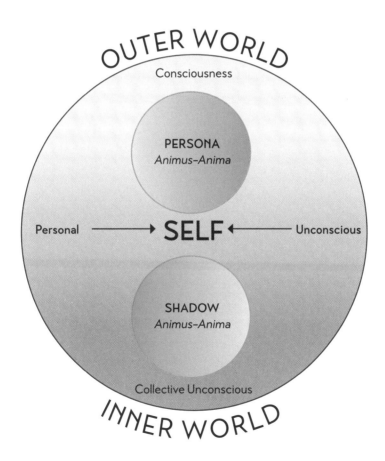

As you can see in the diagram of the self on the previous page, the shadow and the ego exist equal and opposite to each other. The ego is a part of the outer world, and the shadow is a part of the inner world. Our personal unconscious lies beneath our consciousness, and the collective unconscious is buried even deeper beneath that. Jung believed that our conscious mind was not the whole self, and that to achieve true wholeness, each person must go through the process of integrating the shadow aspect. He called this process *individuation*. The method of individuation is where we confront our unconscious elements in order to integrate them into our conscious minds. Once a person begins to acknowledge their persona, which is a social mask that works diligently to hide all their flaws and imperfections, they can then move deeper into integrating the shadow.

Discovering Shadow Work

I discovered shadow work through an extensive self-healing journey I took due to chronic illness symptoms that could not be rectified through Eastern or Western medicine but instead required an extensive multipronged approach to improve my symptoms. Shadow work provided immediate relief from the constant psychic tension I felt after only a few exercises. While my physical symptoms did indeed take longer to remedy, they eventually slowly let up in frequency and severity. I hope that, with enough discovery into the way my mind is programmed, I can reconfigure any flawed data and find absolute relief in the future.

Shadow work has helped me discover so much about myself—and thus has allowed for such deep expansion and profound healing that I've devoted my life to this work. I've committed myself to helping people out of their unconscious painful struggles. I have created online courses and I work with people one-on-one as a coach and counselor in order to effect significant change within a short period of time. It is my dream—and I feel it is my personal mission—to deliver this information to any and all people that it could help. I intuitively perceive that many of the struggles I have personally had to face were the perfect backdrop for a deeper understanding of my shadow education. Since I have lived so much in the dark, I now possess the ability to draw people out of the muck with ample experience and careful guidance.

Contexts in Which Your Shadow Emerges

★ Intense emotional reactions to the behaviors and faults of others
★ Negative feedback (and how you respond to it) regarding your actions and how they affect others
★ Patterns that come up in close relationships and experiences
★ When your impulses overtake your actions
★ Moments where you feel humiliated and embarrassed
★ When traumatic memories and flashbacks come into your awareness

How to Use This Book

This book may be read in any order, although the information does build upon the previous chapters. However, you may start where you feel called. "Consider" questions, "Take Action" boxes, journaling prompts, and activities are suggested and meant to help deepen your understanding. These range from physical activity, such as meditation, to creating artistic images, and of course, a lot of reflective questions that you can use as writing prompts to help you look at things from new perspectives and give you insight into your unconscious aspects and tendencies.

While not required to get the most out of this book, I encourage you to get a journal to work in so that you can write or create when prompted. Many questions will take some time to ponder before an answer comes to your consciousness, so keep these questions in the forefront of your mind until an answer presents itself. You can revisit this book and the activities time and time again to discover more internally and to dig deeper into yourself.

✳   ✳   ✳

1

WHAT IS THE SHADOW?

Understanding the shadow requires a more comprehensive understanding of the ego. The ego is what you strive to be; it is the equivalent of "putting your best foot forward." Broadly, the shadow is essentially the opposite of the ego and everything it deems valuable and worth striving toward. The opposite spectrum of that ego-self is what creates the shadow. This obscure companion has only garnered a bad reputation because of the ego, and all the ways the ego projects its own darkness and evil onto the shadow. Contrary to popular belief, there can also be positive qualities dwelling within the shadow's mysterious depths. The ego doesn't like to look at what it has repressed, so it hides it all from itself. The ego works pretty hard to keep all that is in the shadow concealed.

The thing is, this concealing takes a *lot* of energy from you! Imagine how much energy it takes to hold a beach ball underwater constantly. I told you: it is a lot of work! The ego works diligently to protect you. At least, that's what it is attempting to do because that is its job. The ego needs to recognize itself as good, and when the shadow inadvertently foils this plan, you end up feeling pretty bad psychologically, even if you aren't exactly sure why.

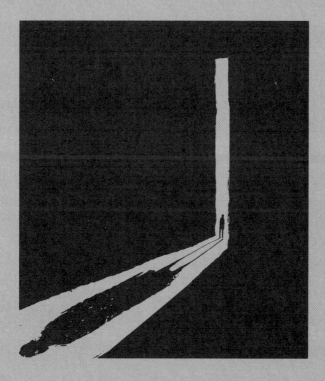

The ego and shadow were created in the same moment, from the same experiences and programming. The creation of the ego cannot occur without the creation of the shadow. It is like yin and yang. One without the other would create a vacuum or a black hole. The shadow works like a psychic immune system, helping to define who and what you are. Different countries, families, cultures, and religions create varying shadows for us all. We each have unique experiences, and what falls into the ego or shadow will depend on what has happened throughout your particular life. Have you ever heard the expression "They carry a lot of emotional baggage"? It is actually quite literal in that most people are carrying around a lot of energy in their shadow.

Okay, so let's imagine you're suppressing essential aspects of your personality because your ego thinks they are undesirable and unacceptable. Can you now imagine holding down another beach ball with the other hand? This one is your trauma and all the ways it has impacted your nervous system, mind, body, and spirit. It sounds challenging to do anything else now, right? You are

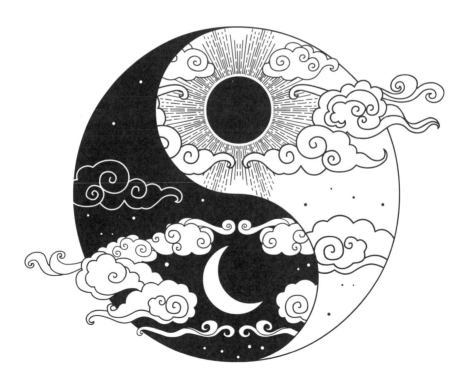

probably feeling extremely drained by all that constant suppression! Wouldn't it be nice to let those beach balls float up to the surface of the water the way nature intended? That's what it's like after you've done some deep digging with shadow work. Suddenly, you have the freedom to exist with complete acceptance of yourself. Just imagine where else you could direct all that energy you are wasting on suppression by trying to please your ego.

What Does It Mean to Be Triggered?

In terms of mental health, a trigger is something that greatly affects your emotional state, often negatively. Triggers are known to cause extreme upset and feelings of being completely overwhelmed with emotion. Those of us who have experienced childhood or ongoing emotional trauma are much more susceptible to reacting to triggers with emotional flashbacks to previous abuse, even when the triggering event seems neutral to an outside observer.

Golden Shadow

The shadow contains positive aspects, even though most people don't realize it. I've come to know these beneficial aspects as the *golden shadow*. The shadow remains connected to the lost parts of our soul, that which makes us human: our creativity and our sense of inspiration. It is difficult to remain open to inspiration if you are closing off large portions of yourself due to internal pain. So, you might ask, what happens to the portions of ourselves we purposely avoid?

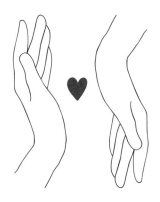

Psychology describes it as *projection*: we project anything buried deep within our own shadow onto others. Golden shadow often arises when we experience an emotion like envy. We were taught we cannot embody that which we are witnessing and actively condemning in another—even if it is an inherent talent or gift within us.

Golden shadow is a perfect example of why it's so pertinent to do shadow work. Someone told you that your unique gifts and talents are not acceptable, and you believed them, even if it meant stuffing a special part of yourself way down into your darkness. Envy is an excellent place to start looking for the golden shadow.

Consider

•••••◆◆◆•••••

★ When do you project your golden shadow?
★ What are the last three times you felt jealous of someone?
★ What is it about them that sparked an intense reaction from you?

Projection: The Roles We Play

Projection is a tool the shadow uses to keep itself hidden. Unknowingly, you project your dark shadow qualities outward onto others. That is why you see shadow indirectly in the traits and actions of other people. The ego tries desperately to keep the shadow outside of yourself. It feels less threatening for the ego to observe it this way. When you experience an intense reaction to another person's behavior, chances are you are projecting your own shadow onto them—thus observing the behavior from a place of repressing energy instead of embodying it.

Looking Closer

We can indirectly explore the roles we play in our own lives by looking at our taste in cinema. These stories on the screen help us to connect with different parts of our repressed selves—especially because we are in a completely relaxed state when we "zone out" and watch these narratives. Over the next few days, try watching some movies and shows that you love. Then move on to watching media with subject matter that you know you don't like as much. Explore all kinds of genres displaying multiple examples of victims, heroes, and villains. Expose yourself to many different storylines to gain a fair representation of

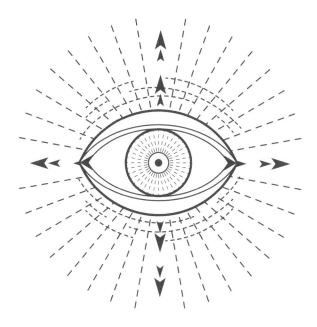

these main archetypal characters. During each TV show or movie, think about the following questions about the characters in the story:

* ★ Which movies light up your shadow and make you feel triggered?
* ★ Which characters do you feel close to?
* ★ Which characters do you love to hate?
* ★ Which characters do you feel sorry for?
* ★ Which characters are you attracted to?
* ★ What kinds of characters make you want to turn off the movie/show?
* ★ Which characters make you want to watch more?

Shadow Soundtrack

Ultimately, the shadow's job is to grab your attention. Think about it: If the shadow threw out subtle hints to you, do you think you would even notice? The shadow exists so deep within your consciousness that it is essentially hiding from you. It takes a conscientious process to uncover what dwells within your unconscious. There are many different approaches to this. Each chapter following this one will be addressing some of the ways to investigate your shadow and process what you come to identify. The more unconscious you are to your shadow side, the darker those fragments of your psyche—mysteriously revealed in extreme stress, intoxication, emotional upset, dreams, and embarrassing moments—will be.

The Impact of Music

Music has such a profound influence on us. I swear, some songs feel like they strike a chord with my very soul. Create a shadow soundtrack to identify with. Songs have the power to transport us to another world—and they can connect us with deeper parts of our psyche, too. Start by exploring different genres of music. Take the time to listen to different types of music from your personal collection and purposefully go beyond your typical listening genres. Push the envelope with what you enjoy and what bothers you, excites you, etc. When you need to tune in to your shadow, make a playlist to get in touch with this part of yourself.

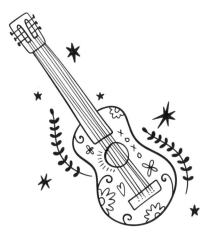

Consider

* What are the most impactful tracks on your shadow soundtrack?
* Make a conscious practice to move to the music and notice how you feel while doing so. How do you feel in your body when you listen? How do you feel emotionally?

Shadow Revealed

No one has ever labeled the process of confronting the shadow as easy or straightforward. Your subconscious mind contains more than just the same primal instincts of your ancestors—even your sense of good and evil stems from here. There is a lot to unpack within this extremely enigmatic shadow self. However, to live a mentally balanced life, you must be diligent about discovering, understanding, and accepting what resides within it, no matter how uncomfortable the integration process might feel at the moment.

So how do we let those beach balls float up to where they rest easily, without the constant pressure to push them deep down under the water? We learn to let them float casually on the surface of our awareness. This same awareness creates an atmosphere where we need not act on impulsive, emotional triggers. Instead, we can recognize them for what they indeed are: a call from your shadow to look at a portion of your psyche that needs integration and healing.

Connecting, Not Conquering

We are so used to pushing the shadow away that when we finally start trying to connect, it is usually quite happy to oblige! Many people think the shadow and the ego are something to conquer or destroy, but they are necessary parts of your consciousness. My approach is to get to know the shadow, accept it, and eventually learn to love it by understanding its conception, thus cultivating compassion for yourself. Starting a frequent conversation with the shadow is a good way to establish a relationship with this part of yourself that is usually quite hidden.

Take Action

★ For ten days in a row, before you begin your day, ask your shadow to reveal itself to you.

★ Keep a journal for each of the moments you get a glimpse of your shadow throughout your day.

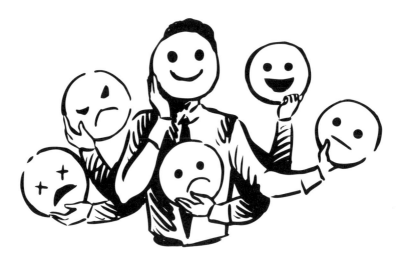

The Masks We Wear

In my own self-discovery of the shadow, I have learned that it is, in fact, a wise teacher with profound ways of initiating one's personal lessons. People would not pay any attention to the shadow without that punch-to-the-gut feeling when it surfaces. My chronic pain taught me to respect the shadow like a wise mentor. You can learn a lot about yourself in discomfort—sometimes much more than you can from contentment. In these moments of agonizing self-reflection, nothing outside of you can affect you or your circumstances. The only solution is to go deep within yourself and find the answers and the keys to unlock the door to freedom.

Your Persona

A persona is a social mask you wear to present yourself to the world. What does your persona reveal about you and your experience in social settings? Let's explore how you project this small version of yourself that you value, rather than the entire "self." We often project this masked version of ourselves because we want to be accepted and loved. So, we try to become someone we deem acceptable and lovable. The thing

Consider

••••◆◆◆◆◆◆◆◆••••

★ In what ways does your persona mask your true self?

★ How could you benefit from dropping your persona?

★ Do you feel confident enough in your authenticity to let down your persona with those you trust?

is, we are much more lovable and enjoyable when we are authentic and true to the nature of our hearts. The more we create a clear understanding of the persona, the more we can recognize and analyze when we are using it, because sometimes we genuinely need it to protect ourselves.

Shadow Image

If you want inner peace, shadow work is definitely a prerequisite. You cannot have a calm and tranquil mind if there is an undercurrent of chaos. The worst part is that since you can't see the undercurrent, you don't even know which direction it is pulling you in. Because of the influence of the ego, most people adamantly avoid uncomfortable thoughts, memories, and feelings. However, they don't disappear; they continue to exist just below our awareness. Within this hidden part of you are the influences that continue to steer you forward in each and every moment of your life. After all, it contains the flawed modeling your parents demonstrated to you with rigorous repetition throughout childhood. It contains embarrassing, awkward moments and primal desires you've deemed shameful. It includes the concepts you learned from your interactions with other people and the traumas that were too painful and destabilizing for you to process in the moment.

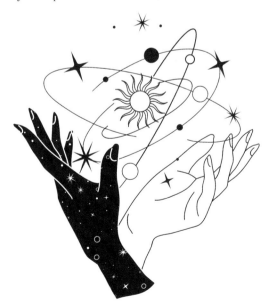

Meditation

Let's take some time to visualize an image of your shadow; this will help to make you more conscious and aware of this part of your psyche. You can use this image in the future when your shadow self is triggering you. By remembering this image and sending your shadow love and appreciation, you are actively integrating it. I strongly suggest practicing this when you are calm and a little sleepy—the more relaxed you are, the better you will be able to connect with your shadow. Remember to acknowledge and thank this unappreciated part of you.

1. Begin by taking a comfortable seat where you won't be distracted. Take three long, deep breaths to center your mind and clear it of all thoughts.

2. Close your eyes and ask your subconscious to bring to mind an image of your shadow. Allow yourself to visualize it in detail, producing a clear picture.

3. Meditate on this for five minutes. Notice what you are shown. Sit with the image in your mind and become comfortable with it.

4. Note how you feel when you visualize the image you created. Does it make you anxious? Afraid? Maybe you're feeling a little uncomfortable. Or possibly you feel some emotional relief at having recognized it. Remember this image so that you can conjure it later, anytime you need it.

5. Imagine that you're wrapping your arms around your shadow with full acceptance and love for it. Hold this visual and really feel the love that you're giving it.

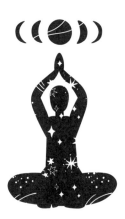

6. Take three deep breaths to close the practice, then slowly open your eyes and adjust back into the physical world.

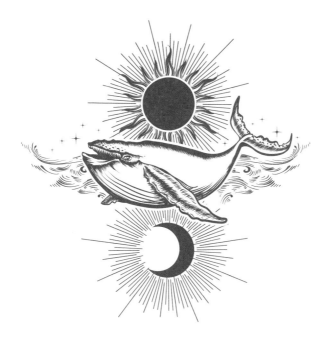

Once you develop an awareness of your own unconscious aspects of the psyche, the shadow begins to take on an identifiable form. That is how we practice shadow work: creating form out of the formless through deeper and deeper recognition of your psyche. Ultimately, shadow work is a psychological process of self-realization on all levels. It is the process of integrating unconscious aspects of the psyche into your conscious awareness to live a more mentally balanced life. It is essential to examine the programming you have received throughout your life, especially in childhood. It's important to take a deep dive into your subconscious mind to look at what might be triggering emotional reactions to current situations. Seeing things more clearly will enable you to avoid future projections of your fears and insecurities. When you learn how to move through your life with total awareness, you will discover unlimited power and grace within you.

Now that you have successfully begun to create a sense of your shadow, make sure to continue to utilize these techniques to stay in touch with it—that way, your shadow has a line of open communication with you. It does not need to trigger you with cataclysmic mishaps to gain your attention. I know that triggers are unpleasant, so let's try to avoid them as much as possible by staying in conscious contact with the shadow.

❋ ❋ ❋

2

WHAT IS SHADOW WORK?

In the previous chapter, we discussed what the shadow is—but what is shadow work? What does that even mean? Shadow work is all the ways we confront the unconscious aspects of ourselves and how we process and integrate the information that we discover. So, how do we do that? First, we must discover what we've hidden from ourselves for fear of disappointing our family. Rejection is painful. The brain reacts to rejection like physical pain. No wonder we spend a great deal of energy avoiding it. Here's the thing though: You can't be authentic or vulnerable (two very worthwhile endeavors) without risking rejection. Really? Yes, it's true! Think about it: How can I authentically be myself without also risking that you may not like who I am? The shadow is actively covering up and hiding everything that might cause you to feel rejected. Why? Because those things are hard to look at, deal with, and understand. The shadow's job is to conceal things until a trigger shows us where to integrate, so that's exactly what it will do: *trigger you.* So, you might ask, "Why should I go digging up old junk?" Well, if you want to become your true authentic self, you have to understand where you're limiting yourself and wasting precious energy on projection and repression.

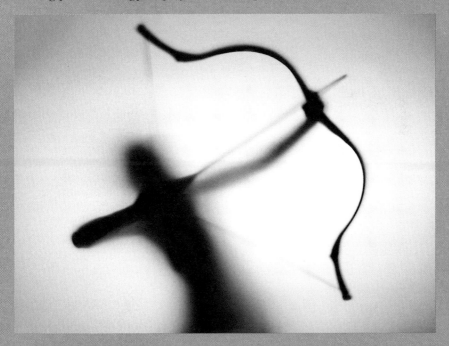

Using shadow work, you will begin to look at the world and the people in it very differently. You will gain so much understanding just by making a rapid assessment of their internal workings. Because, when you know how to look for them, they are all displayed outwardly in one way or another. When you witness cycles in people that you just can't understand—for instance, how some choose to harm themselves with irrational decisions over and over—that is their shadow playing out a pattern. A lot of people in the world are still suffering the effects of the traumas they experienced. When the nervous system is dysregulated, it is easy to make poor choices and seek out familiar territory like abusive situations. Without this insight some just think they have bad luck—as the saying goes, "that's the cards they were dealt." In all reality, the repeated pattern of an uncomfortable or emotionally abusive situation may be led by their unconscious. Shadow work is a process of taking the time to really know yourself intimately. Question everything, then make time to question everything all over again, including the conclusions you have already realized.

Okay, so how do we actually do it? How does one turn on a light in a dark room? There are infinite ways. We are here to create form out of formlessness, so we will do some out-of-the-box thinking where you learn to pin down your elusive shadow, if only for a moment. These questions and activities will help you discover ways to invite this new friend into your daily routine, and into your thoughts and feelings.

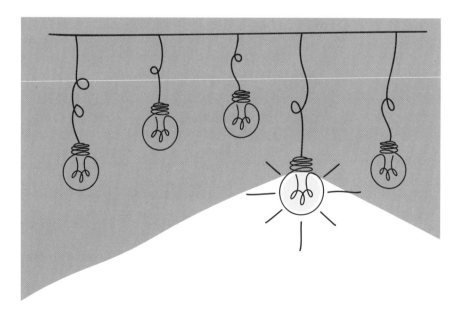

What Are Some of the Benefits of Doing Shadow Work?

★ Achieve more self-acceptance, not of your projected ego-self but of your authentic personality and interests
★ Handle emotional upheaval with a clear head and balanced reactions
★ Feel less intense reactions to emotional triggers
★ Free yourself from unnecessary and unwarranted guilt and shame
★ Recognize your projections rather than misplacing negative energy onto others, allowing you to heal inwardly
★ Maintain healthy relationships with honest, open communication and frequent self-examination
★ Access the unlimited creativity and potential of your mind
★ Moments where you feel humiliated and embarrassed
★ When traumatic memories and flashbacks come into your awareness

Light and Dark Aspects

The shadow is frequently a theme in mythology and literature as the battle between two siblings or twins, one good and one evil. These twins symbolize the dual nature of the universe and the light and dark sides of consciousness: the ego and the alter ego. When combined, the siblings form a whole—just like when we work to integrate the shadow, we move closer to wholeness. In some ways, shadow work is like chasing your tail. There will always be a chase. It will never be "caught." There is always something new to be illuminated. Another analogy is that it's like a dance: Take one step forward, then inevitably two steps backward, but the dance continues.

Amazingly, the shadow seems to be something not only hidden from our consciousness but hidden from society as well. In my opinion, I believe when we learn of these characters in literature and mythology, the shadow aspect should be explained so we can collectively move toward conscious awareness. Let's unpack this mythological theme further by exploring the sibling (or sibling-like) relationships that you have had experience with.

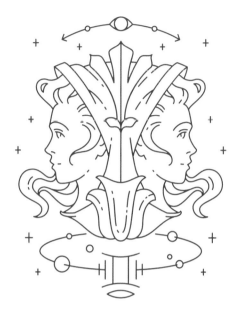

Consider

* Think about a relationship between two siblings or twins that you know. In what ways do these siblings represent polar opposites of one another?
* Do you have a close friend that you feel is like your sibling? What do you think is the benefit of having a person to foster opposition in such close proximity to you?
* Has your shadow ever revealed itself with this friend?
* Can you see your shadow in this friend? (For example, do they do things that you judge harshly? Do they aggravate you in certain ways?)

The False Self

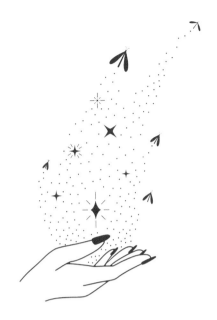

During the creation of the shadow, we create three separate aspects of the self to deal with the pain of repression and to splinter it further away from our conscious awareness. First, we have the False Self—a version of ourselves we made to fill the void created by repression and inadequate nurturing. We created the False Self to be liked and accepted by our caretakers, to fit in, and to reserve our seat at the proverbial table.

Looking Closer

Children are physiologically very delicate and dependent upon the love and generosity of their caregivers. If they are rejected by those with moral obligations to see to their safety, they could be gravely harmed. So even though we are wired to connect with others from birth, our authentic nature comes second to our need for approval. This is why the shadow is created: to protect the child by hiding the parts that are not accepted and approved of by the parents. Childhood is much less painful this way, but eventually, if we desire to be whole and integrated, these repressed and undesirable aspects must be accepted.

- ★ What happened when you didn't behave the way your caretakers desired?
- ★ As a result, how did you modify your behaviors to please them?
- ★ List the five most impactful times you ever felt rejected.
- ★ How did these moments mold you into a false version of yourself?
- ★ What did you internalize from these moments of rejection?
- ★ In what ways are you still protecting yourself from being rejected in the same way?

The Disowned Self

Next, we have the Disowned Self—parts of the False Self that were disapproved of and then denied to foster acceptance. Frequently these are negative aspects of the False Self. The ego will always generate a Disowned Self because we naturally disown that which does not fit into the developing picture of who we think we are. The ego cultivates a one-sided nature, meaning our neglected, rejected, and unacceptable qualities accumulate in the unconscious. These qualities take the form of an inferior personality. What is "disowned" does not "disappear"; it lives on in our psyche. Out

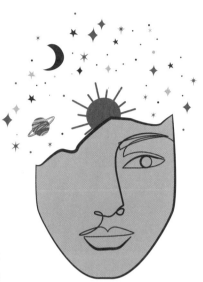

Take Action

★ Ask yourself: What am I actively suppressing that I don't consciously know about? Over the course of the next ten days, keep this question fresh in your mind and let the answers come to you. Jot down your realizations.

★ For each one, ask yourself: How does suppressing this part of myself actually benefit me? Is it truly benefiting me, or is my ego just trying to convince me of that to try to protect itself?

★ If you stopped suppressing these, what would embodying them look and feel like?

★ From the instances where you were rejected for displaying your False Self, take note of which behaviors or characteristics were rejected by others and write them down to revisit later, as you grow.

of sight but not out of mind, a real alter ego always hides just below our level of conscious awareness, erupting when we least expect it due to overwhelming emotional circumstances.

While the False Self may have some positive characteristics, the Disowned Self is the negative portion of that False Self that was created due to further rejection. These negative behaviors or characteristics are rejected by our caretakers and our community, so we disown them to remain likable and socially acceptable. It's important to differentiate these various aspects of self so that we can actively work on bringing them back into our conscious awareness and acceptance.

The Lost Self

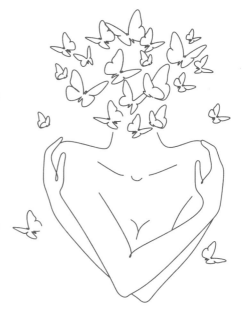

Last, we have the Lost Self. These are the parts of your being that you had to repress because of the demands of society. The Lost Self is a part of you that was lost in the creation of the ego and shadow. It is an aspect of your true nature that you were forced to deny due to societal undercurrents and pressures. You will notice that the False Self and the Disowned Self are portions of the psyche that you are using to cover up the real you out of fear of rejection. However, the Lost Self was a real part of you that was shown to others and, unfortunately, rejected.

I think the Lost Self is the most painful. With the False Self and Disowned Self, we are essentially making up a self that would foster appreciation from others; however, the Lost Self was not a façade but a real aspect we shared in vulnerability and for which we were rejected. Ouch. Let's work on rekindling this Lost Self and garner a new appreciation for its wonderful existence. We must cultivate self-love for this part of us and mourn the time we've spent hiding such a delicate piece of our inner landscape. What are some of the most restrictive demands that society puts on you, and why do you feel it's necessary to adhere to those standards? Think of someone, either a friend, family member, or even a celebrity, who seems to live out loud despite social norms. How do they conduct themselves and make it work for them? Taking example from those we trust or look up to is one way to get started.

Patterns Play Out

Trauma makes rejection feel extremely scary because we've already experienced what it feels like to be rejected (the trauma) and it's gut-wrenching. Not only is it cognitively disruptive, but it also physically impacts the mind and body. Trauma continues to take control of our nervous system until the brain can relax and the threat is determined to be resolved. For some people, this resolution never happens. In an abusive environment, the threats are ongoing, and our personalities and behaviors are shaped by the constant need for regulation.

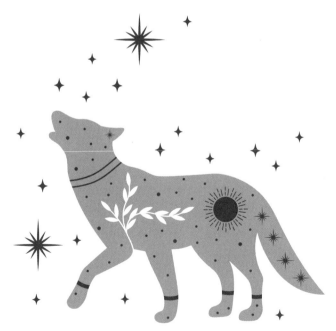

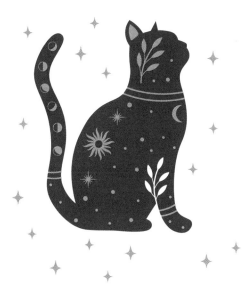

Looking Closer

Nervous system regulation looks different in every household, and in some, it's sparse or nonexistent. I want you to think back to your childhood environment and ponder the dynamics that you were exposed to as you grew up. As humans, we seek out familiarity and inevitably play out some of the same patterns we witnessed as children. Taking a look at the past and identifying the similarities it shares with your life now can help you recognize when you are surrounding yourself with toxic nostalgia.

* ★ What was the overall tone of your household and who set it?
* ★ Who sets the tone of your life now?
* ★ Were your caretakers strict or laid-back?
* ★ Do you find comfort in being strict with yourself now? Or do you prefer to be more laid-back?
* ★ How do you feel about leaning a bit more into the opposite approach? In what ways could this benefit you?
* ★ What about your romantic partners? What patterns do you notice?
* ★ What do you prefer with them?

Conscious Connection

We all have some kind of trauma, even if it's just the trauma of separation from our creator at birth. Healing is really about allowing yourself the space to witness the trauma for what it is without an attachment to what you think should have happened. In this separation, you can process a subtle realization that maybe some piece of this moment unlocked access to another level of growth—but only after you find the meaning behind the pain. There are always lessons from pain. Shadow work is grabbing a shovel and digging to find them.

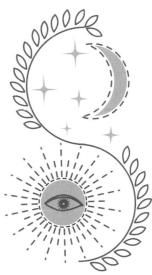

In case you haven't noticed, you live in a paradoxical universe, filled with many different variations of reality. The light and the dark dance back and forth like a candle flame flickering in the darkness of the night. If you believe in a higher power, perhaps you'll see this dance as proof of that higher power's existence. Perhaps you'll see it as proof of chaos and that there is no order—only disorder. For me personally, I find it difficult to believe such an intricate dance between dark and light could ever be coincidental.

Consider

★ Think about a moment where you felt really connected to the source (aka the universe, God, nature, family, or yourself). What did these moments teach you?

★ Think about a moment where you felt really disconnected and lost. What did it feel like?

★ What are some impactful moments where you felt like you were an outsider? What are some moments where you felt included?

It's no wonder we try to disown these uncomfortable bits and pieces of our psyche; they're difficult to process and difficult to understand, but necessary if you want to stop burying a large part of yourself under your coping mechanisms. Emotional maturity is so rare, but it is so necessary for the evolution of humanity. On the world stage, you will see adults behaving just like children, some of whom are the very people making decisions that control our collective fate. Fear and hate for everyone different from you is shadow projection: The more we repress, the more we regress to a childlike mental state where our cognitive dissonance will block out any conflict with what we already believe to be true.

Facing the Darkness

Spiritual growth looks different for everyone, but eventually, you're going to have to face your darkness. If you don't know what to do when it surfaces, you'll be utterly dismayed, even horrified. It will feel out of control and chaotic. You won't understand its presence, and you'll be shocked by its very existence. Up until our individual discovery of our personal shadow, we spend a great deal of our time living in a fantasy that we are "good" and don't have any "bad" within us. This is just plain untrue, and the proper dismantling of trying to judge yourself and others as "good" or "bad" must be accomplished.

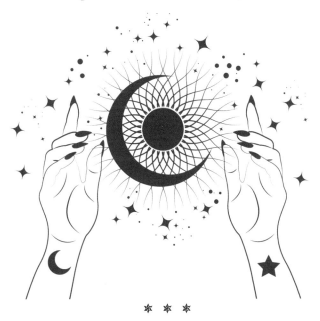

✳ ✳ ✳

3

THE HERO'S JOURNEY

Pain is an exceptional motivator, and the hero's journey is the ultimate catalyst for growth. It will catapult you into a broader experience—one where you reach a deeper awareness of your life's true purpose. If we didn't have pain to teach us, would we ever pay attention to the call of our soul? Many people who feel called to practice shadow work are often on a hero's journey. This journey is more significant than a personal calling to heal and can be more like an ancestral line's yearning for a family member to break generational curses.

I have learned that certain yogic traditions believe that the inner work we do on ourselves to reach enlightenment trickles down seven generations into our past and future. Ancestral DNA is running through your blood now. Are you succumbing to its influence? Or are you influencing it to evolve? From a greater perspective, you will begin to see your individual healing journey as an opportunity to sever ancestral traumas that would continue to live on in future generations without your careful dismantling of these oppressive internal systems. This chapter will weave the pattern of your own personal hero's journey into the tapestry of your family's heroic lineage and allow you to carefully consider all that your ancestors have overcome to create the fortuitous opportunity of your very existence.

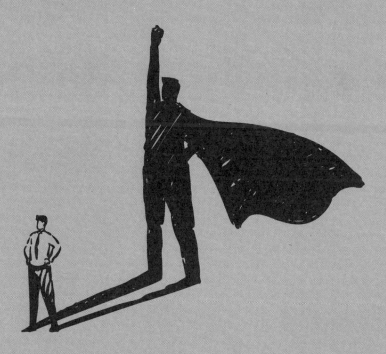

The shadow is created to shelter us from pain, but pain is inevitable. Since we can all agree on its inevitability, perhaps we can learn to accept its presence without fear. In no way do I mean to glorify pain; I merely accept that I will experience it from time to time. After all, it is just a sensation like any other: It is the labels and judgments we place upon it that give it such immense power. Pain holds within it the gift of knowledge and experience. Your capacity to feel pain is equal and opposite to your capacity to feel joy and expansion. If you can't hold either extreme, you will be living a dull existence. Pain makes living feel like you're walking on a razor's edge. Without it, imagine what the human experience would look like. People would be constantly crashing into each other, both physically and emotionally, to feel something. Boundaries wouldn't exist, and we would all bleed together. Pain creates edges for us to exist within.

Love is borderless, but pain indeed has boundaries. Within the dark magic that is pain exists a liquid alchemical nectar—a medicine. The pain that brings you to your knees contains the same medicine that allows you to stand strong in the face of adversity. The strength it takes to endure the pain is the antivenom that makes you that much more unshakable once you transmute the dark energy. Pain stretches you into a new version of yourself, expanding your capability to hold energy and direct it toward your will. You cannot avoid this wise teacher, because in its avoidance a great measure of your power is lost.

Breakdown or Breakthrough?

In Western culture, pain is avoided as if life depends on it, but it is in this very medicine—when taken by the spoonful rather than the bucket—that real alchemical treasure resides. Without these initiations into a more advanced level of the game that is life, we tend to live at a very surface level. Pain is a thread that connects us all; the different colors and textures create the tapestry that makes each of us unique. Each new layer of the design gives us a deeper understanding of our ultimate purpose. More advanced designs hold within them a greater depth, and they are infinitely more valuable.

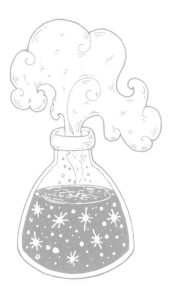

Let's explore the painful moments in your life to make sure we are extracting the precious medicine that exists there. It is only by careful reflection that we grow from pain rather than succumb to it. Pain holds an equal and opposite treasure inside of it: the growth that is possible due to its very existence. Without pain, growth is not possible. Have you ever heard the term "growing pains"? It's quite literal.

Consider

·····◆◆◆◆◆◆·····

★ What would you consider to be the three darkest periods of your life?
★ Did any big doors or opportunities open for you after you made it through?
★ What did you learn about yourself from these times?
★ What growth occurred in their aftermath?

A hero's journey is one met with
many dark nights of the soul because
the hero must be developed. At the
beginning of the story, the hero is not
a hero—just a normal person, neither
brave nor strong. The hero is molded
by the journey and the darkness they
encounter. Each trial and tribulation
tests their resolve, inevitably making
them stronger and more capable with
each hurdle that is passed without
relinquishment. Sometimes those
moments we've been through still
linger in the back of our minds.
Though just below the surface of
our consciousness, they still influence
us greatly.

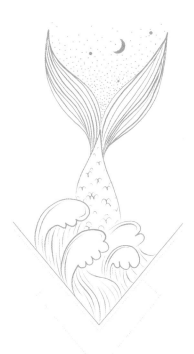

Repetition and Reprogramming

Traumatic memories are influencing your nervous system and letting your
body know it is not yet safe to relax and let your guard down. If you've
experienced enough trauma, whether physical or emotional, your body won't
ever get the signal that it's all right to relax now. This can cause a lot of
issues later down the line. Let's work on reprogramming. I want to stress
the importance of repetition. I invite you to meditate and visualize a difficult
situation and the outcome you *wish* took place, rather than the unsatisfactory
way that it happened. Practice this over and over in a relaxed state. With
this visualization, you are reprogramming the memory in your brain. Try
one memory five times; keep track in your journal. After you've completed
reprogramming, come back and notice how the emotional charge has shifted
when you think about the same memory. You can do this with any negative
memory, but repetition is the key.

Personal Hero's Journey

What makes the hero's journey worthwhile? I'm not exactly sure, but there is just something so completely human about using the power of your own heart to endure great adversities. From what I can tell, that's just how this world works; duality is its blueprint. Without each side of the spectrum readily available to experience, we are left with mundane, boring possibilities, even if comfort is abundant.

Looking Closer

I want you to define what a hero is in your eyes. It's imperative that you celebrate your own strength and countless victories. We live in a challenging environment; honestly, mere survival is applaudable. Happiness, security, and contentment seem like unattainable goals for some. I hope to inspire some gratitude for that which you have already accomplished and praise you for all the benefits you will bring to this world by integrating your shadow.

Answer the following questions in your journal and revisit them often:

* ★ What do you think makes you a hero?
* ★ List three events where you acted heroically.
* ★ How have these events made you more of a hero?
* ★ Draw some of your superpowers in your journal.
* ★ How can you applaud your own victories more often?
* ★ How can you show up feeling like a hero every day?

Ancestors' Legacies

Testing one's will against all odds makes us feel like we are truly alive. We're immersing ourselves in the human experience, even though it's messy and unpredictable. The hero's journey is archetypal because we as humans can all relate to it. We all have some kind of battle we're fighting at one time or another. What does that tell you about human nature and our capabilities? It

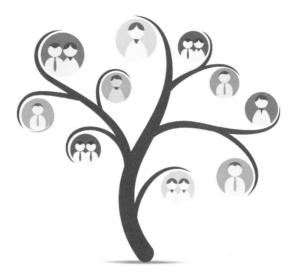

tells me we are willing to test ourselves in order to grow and develop. What a miraculous gift for a species! Could you imagine if we stayed content in our comfort and withered into oblivion?

We all fight battles. Your ancestors fought countless battles just so you would have the opportunity to exist. Did you know you have roughly a billion ancestors? This absolutely boggles my mind. Can you imagine the struggles that your ancestors had to survive just to create you? You have all that ancestral knowledge running through your bloodstream right now. Imagine how much power is lying dormant there.

Consider

* What do you know about your ancestors?
* What are some of the most profound stories you've heard about your family?
* What do you know about your ancestral trauma?
* In what ways has the trauma been passed down?
* If these generational traumas were to be broken, what would that look like?

Lineage of Heroes

Just as we have a lot of dormant power residing in our DNA, we also have an incredible amount of shadow and trauma that has inevitably been passed down. Many of our ancestors did not have access to the tools we have for maintaining a healthy state of mind. Mental health advocacy the way we know it today is something fairly new, and I know for my parents and grandparents who suffered their own childhood traumas that this type of awareness wasn't typical. When we don't have any treatments for or resolutions to trauma, it lives on in the experiencer and inevitably is passed down to their offspring. Humanity made it through these periods with a lot of natural nervous system regulators and a strong connection to our families and communities.

It's crucial to realize we all have pain and trauma passed down our lineage; it helps us dismantle toxic systems. We also need to understand that our ancestors did the best with the tools they had at the time. We have such a better opportunity to heal family systems with our current access to so much information and healing resources. Sometimes the hero is the one who has to bring the family through the dark times.

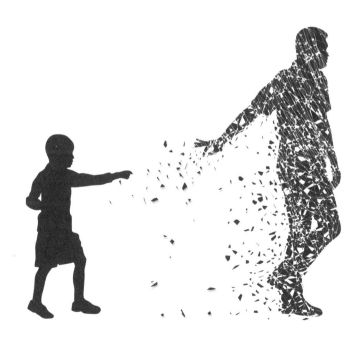

The Family Scapegoat

Family members inevitably bring out shadows in one another. The scapegoat of the family is the one who decided to take on the shadow of the entire ancestry. They are the ones working hard to dismantle toxic family systems. This is no easy task, and the scapegoat pays the price with a lot of darkness passed down from generations that they need to work through. The reason that they are rejected by the rest of the family is because the scapegoat is a mirror of the family's shadow, and it's uncomfortable to be around.

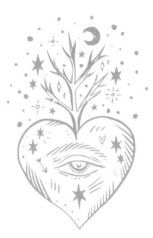

I think visualization is such a powerful tool for the mind to find a resolution. It amazes me that when we cannot find a real-life resolution to our relationships, our brains can also accept the substitute of imagining it yourself. We took the time to reprogram some of our trauma; we will now do the same with your family lineage.

Take Action

······◆◆◆◆◆◆◆······

★ I want you to imagine and then describe in detail your family thriving in a healthy way in your journal. Describe what that would look like and feel like.

★ I invite you to meditate and visualize the way you wish it were. Practice this over and over in a relaxed state. You are essentially reprogramming your brain. Try one visualization ten times and keep track in your journal.

★ After you've completed reprogramming, write about how you feel now when you think of your family.

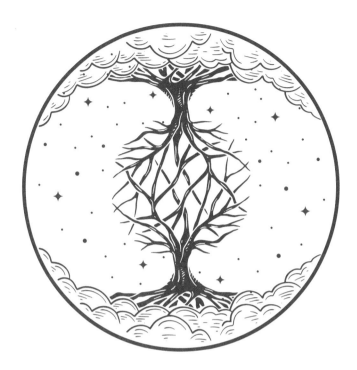

I hope this chapter has allowed you to look at your personal hero's journey from a broader perspective. You now understand the context of your pain as it relates to your personal story, and how you come from a long history of heroes overcoming countless adversities for you to have the life you live today. Do you feel like you are a hero from a lineage of heroes? Well, you are—we all are. We all share the same ancestors when you go back far enough, and we all have the same stories at some point in our history. We share the same blood; we are all interconnected and interwoven by our shared humanity. A large part of that humanity is lost in the shadow. We each have one, but we all share a collective shadow as well. We are all just mirrors for one another so that we can integrate and heal. What a beautiful paradox.

Don't be afraid to tell the story of your existence. Integrate your family's story and yours together, interwoven like they truly are; separation is merely a flawed perception. I want you to really know how heroic you are and how you were born from heroes who survived against all odds just so that you could come to this planet to take a breath.

✳ ✳ ✳

4

THE UNCONSCIOUS, SUBCONSCIOUS, AND CONSCIOUS MIND

Your mind communicates through neurons in the brain, which produce synchronized electrical impulses called brain waves. When masses of neurons communicate with one another, they generate brain waves in a range of frequencies. Some of these cycle rapidly, and some slowly. These brain waves influence your level of consciousness. Out of the three levels of consciousness, the conscious mind is what you know best. This is your basic day-to-day thinking state: your normal problem-solving and thought-processing state you experience when awake and alert. The brain waves in this state are called beta and gamma. This is the state where you have conscious access to the frontal lobe—aka the thinking and processing region of your brain—and can easily process incoming information. Alpha waves are slower and represent a state of relaxation and idleness where the brain waits on hold, responding when needed. This is the subconscious mind, the layer beneath the conscious mind. We are aware of what exists here, but for the moment it is outside of our awareness. Every imprint you've experienced in your life is kept here: Every thought, every word you've spoken or heard, every memory, and every feeling is kept as if in a database or hard drive. When you drive home but aren't actually thinking about how to get there, you can thank the subconscious mind for that. In other words, your subconscious is your second nature, or autopilot part of the mind.

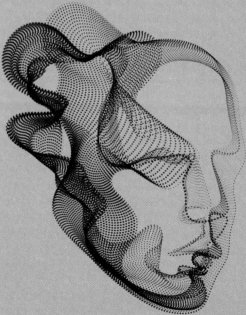

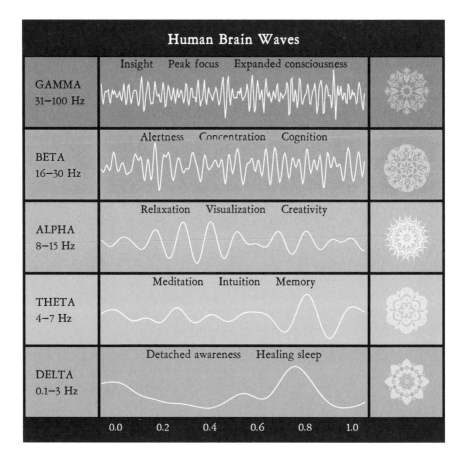

Now let's talk about the last level of consciousness, the unconscious mind. This is represented by the theta and delta waves, the slowest frequency brain waves. Theta is a dreamlike state similar to a daydream or a trance, while delta is the deepest dream state that we experience during REM sleep cycles. The unconscious mind is where some memories are actively kept hidden from your consciousness, such as traumatic, painful memories, and any imprints formed up until approximately seven years old (before beta brain waves became dominant). This is where your beliefs, behaviors, patterns, attitudes, and habits are. While the conscious mind can easily recall information from the subconscious mind, it cannot recall information from the unconscious mind without deep meditative states or hypnosis. These trancelike states quiet the conscious mind, which allows access through the gateway of our unconscious mind.

Subconscious Desire

We all think we are running the show with our conscious mind, but we are not. The thing about the subconscious mind is that its subtle influence is actually the steward of our human vessel. Our brain is actively using all the information stored in the subconscious to try to protect us from getting hurt physically or emotionally. This is because when we're in emotional pain, the brain equates this feeling to physical pain.

Your conscious mind is the state of mind you are familiar with, but did you know a great deal of your thought process is directed by the subconscious and unconscious minds? Science just doesn't understand exactly how yet, but scientists are beginning to do more research. If a great deal of your mind's capacity is being utilized by the parts that are not conscious to you, you can begin to understand how the subconscious is the captain that is steering your "vessel."

Whenever you get a result that you are disappointed in, I implore you to consider these four questions:

1. In what way did I expect this outcome?
2. In what way did I desire this outcome?
3. In what way do I agree with this outcome?
4. What is my subconscious belief about this outcome?

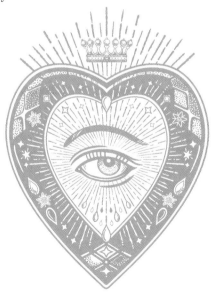

Stream of Subconsciousness

If your brain is using every bit of information it's ever received to try to keep you from getting hurt again, can you see where some problems might arise? Your brain will tell you, "Stay in your comfort zone" or "Stay safe" when that might not actually be in your best interest. You might waste your talent and innate gifts by not using them because your brain tells you it's dangerous, especially if you have trauma. Trauma impacts the subconscious mind tremendously, and as you'll learn later in this book, it takes a great deal of work to untangle the threads that connect us to our trauma.

Have you ever tried stream-of-consciousness writing or journaling? It's a great way to let your subconscious mind flow and get some of the junk out of the way. Something about it is very cathartic. Let's do a subconscious mind dump and see what your subconscious is trying to tell you. Start by meditating for five minutes. I'll show you an easy meditation that you can use for this, and for any time you feel triggered—it will help you calm down within three minutes of continued practice.

★ **MEDITATE FOR FIVE MINUTES:** Start by closing your eyes and inhaling slowly while counting to five. Try to match your breath with the amount of time it takes you to count. Now hold your breath in for the count of five. Exhale as slowly as possible while you count to seven. Pause for a moment with the breath held out, then inhale again. Repeat for five minutes. Bonus points if you set the ambience to get even more relaxed: soft music, dim lighting, a clean space, an inviting scent, etc.

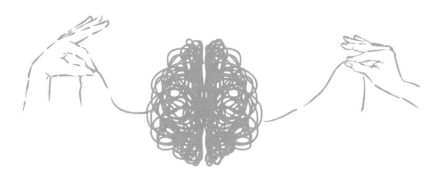

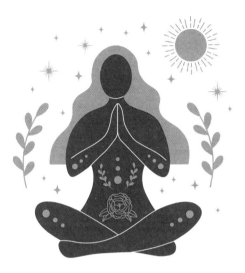

★ **FLOW:** After meditating, sit down and, with a clear mind, ask your subconscious to communicate with you via journaling. Allow a stream of consciousness to just flow through you. Fill up the blank space.

★ **READ IT BACK:** What did you learn about your subconscious after reading?

★ **REPEAT:** Continue this practice for one week. Jot down anything important that comes into your awareness.

Subconscious Language

You are beginning to realize the power of your subconscious mind. You are becoming aware that this mysterious part of your mind subtly directs your entire life; everything you say and do is because of the direction of your subconscious. This means that you can go through a lifetime of therapy and work painstakingly on improving yourself, but all your efforts will be with your conscious mind. If you never deal with your shadow, your life will still be driven by your subconscious. No matter how much effort you expend, you will self-sabotage your valiant efforts without even realizing it. You won't be able to see how your unconscious thoughts, beliefs, and behaviors have contributed to your missteps.

Looking Closer

Think of it almost like a car driving down the highway with no one at the wheel—just someone in the back seat who is spouting vague directions in the form of symbols, feelings, and images. I used to have a recurring dream where suddenly I was in a car and I was supposed to be driving, but I was not in the driver's seat. Now I can finally understand the cryptic symbolism. Let's try speaking to the subconscious in its own language:

★ Think about an intention. Hold this intention in your mind as you create an abstract image using shapes and symbols that reflect it on a piece of paper.

★ Now allow your only intention to be for your subconscious mind to communicate with you. Ask your subconscious a question and ask it to draw out an answer for you using shapes and symbols or whatever you are directed to.

★ Look at the image and translate it. What does it mean?

★ Now ask your subconscious to communicate with you about anything you should be aware of at this time. Ask your subconscious to draw an image of this information.

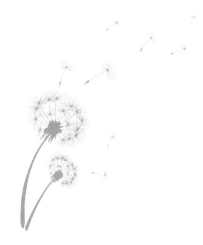

★ After you've drawn it, what do you see? What does this message mean?

What Imprints Are You Creating?

It's important to understand that your thoughts and actions make up your self-concept; they are the foundation the conscious mind stands upon. So, if your subconscious thoughts and beliefs are that you aren't good enough to accomplish what you desire, your subconscious will make sure you don't follow through. This happens because the subconscious has a confirmation bias, protecting you by creating a reality in which its beliefs are proven correct. Now can you see how this "protection" can be holding you back from the life you actually want?

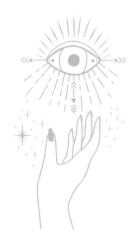

So how do we escape the limitations our own subconscious mind has put upon us? By reprogramming the information that is not useful or even true. All that junk that was implanted by your family, school, the media, and your peers needs to be altered because it is flawed, and most of it doesn't actually benefit you whatsoever. More often than not, it actively tears your confidence down and makes you insecure, depressed, and anxious. We must reprogram this faulty information by changing the narrative and creating our own—one that is true and takes into consideration our unlimited possibilities and the power of our will to break through limitations and preconceived barriers. What are you currently putting into your subconscious mind?

Consider

* ★ What movies and shows do you watch?
* ★ How much news do you consume?
* ★ What books are you reading?
* ★ Are these imprints helping you to feel good?
* ★ Is there anything you should stop consuming unconsciously?

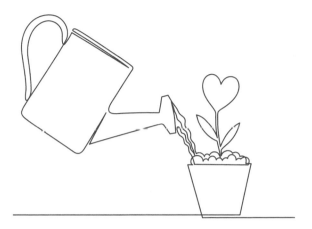

Unconscious Clues

You might be thinking, "Why would anyone want to access the unconscious mind?" If you have childhood trauma or traumatic memories that need to be reprogrammed, you will need to access this part of your consciousness to do so. However, one must be careful tapping into this aspect because you can also do damage if you aren't aware of the impact this will have on you. If you have significant trauma (like severe emotional, physical, or sexual abuse), I always recommend that you see a therapist or counselor when accessing these memories and be prepared to face the emotional ups and downs that will accompany digging up what you've previously buried. Make sure you are in a very healthy mental state before attempting to access painful memories.

Accessing the Subconscious Mind

You will know when you are ready to go that deep, but first, you must break down the initial layers of shadow before access is available. For now, we will access the unconscious mind through inkblots. What you see in these abstract shapes will give you some insight into your unconscious mind and what it is trying to express to you. If nothing comes to mind, try coming back in a relaxed state—after a bath, right before bed, or upon awakening. You can practice this repeatedly to test the undercurrent of your unconscious mind.

What do you see in this image? How does it make you feel? What thoughts does it cause you to think? What does this tell you about your unconscious mind?

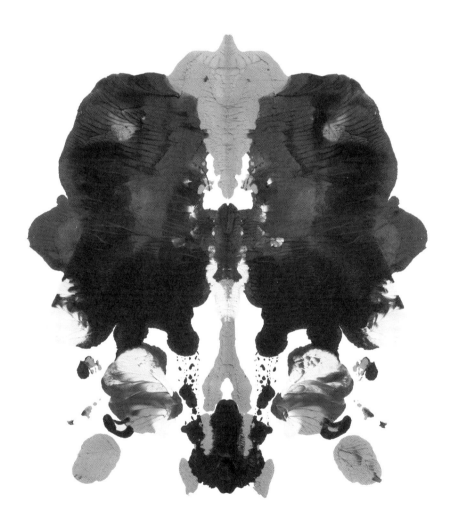

What do you see in this image? How does it make you feel? What thoughts does it cause you to think? What does this tell you about your unconscious mind?

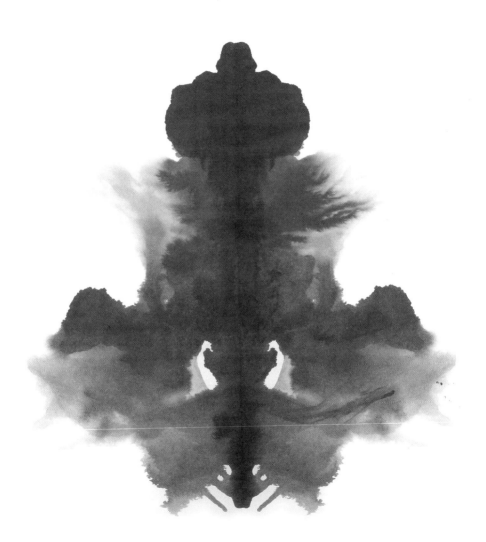

What do you see in this image? How does it make you feel? What thoughts does it cause you to think? What does this tell you about your unconscious mind?

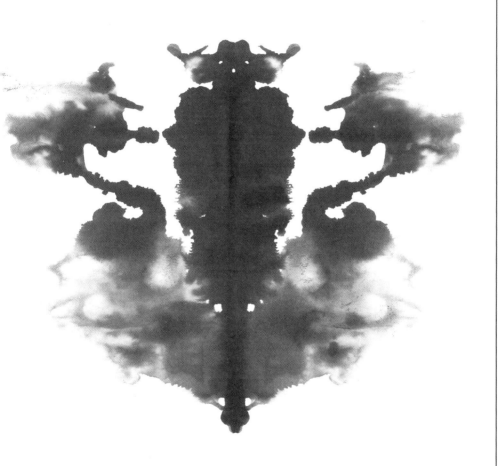

Rapid Transformational Therapy

Another way to access your subconscious mind is through Rapid Transformational Therapy. Working with this technique helps you get into the brain wave state needed to access the subconscious. Once you can effectively communicate with this aspect of yourself, you can begin to see where you need

Take Action

Find new ways to use creativity to communicate with the levels of consciousness below your awareness. Try new approaches to use your creative side. Don't be judgmental about what you do or create; just allow creativity to flow through you and enjoy the moment. Continue the practice of what you enjoy the most and make a commitment to keep doing it.

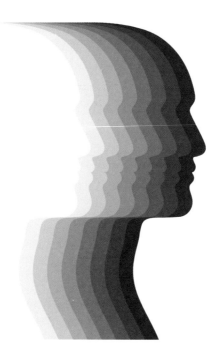

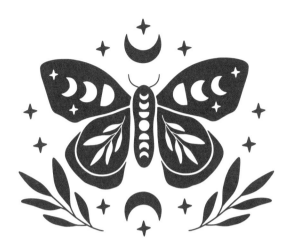

healing and start shifting your negative beliefs, even about yourself. A session of RTT with a trained therapist will walk you through psychotherapy, neuro-linguistic programming, cognitive behavioral therapy, and your own memories to target your core beliefs, emotions, and value systems. This throws the doors of the subconscious wide open, giving you insight into things that have been long buried within you.

What's the point of accessing this info and reprogramming it? I guess the question is: Do you want to have some control over the path you are heading down? Well, as I mentioned, if you don't influence the subconscious mind with information that is useful and beneficial to you, you will constantly be at the mercy of your programming from childhood and thus far. Real, significant changes in a person's life shift from the subconscious mind first, and then the change happens in the conscious mind after the fact.

Take the time to consciously reprogram your most potent traumatic memories, because these memories influence you in every moment. Give your mind a resolution: Due to the way procedural memories are formed, which is when repeated signals are reinforced between synapses, we have the ability to reprogram our minds with repetition. So, your act of visualizing the scenario you desire is reprogramming your consciousness. The important part is to do this over and over. Repetition helps new programming further influence the subconscious.

❊   ❊   ❊

5

THE INNER CHILD NEEDS HEALING

We were all children once, and now that childlike aspect still lives on within us. Psychology has deemed the inner child a genuine part of our psyche. In fact, most behavioral, emotional, and relationship issues are known to stem from here. Hopefully, you are beginning to understand what a profound impact your childhood experiences have had on your current reality due to the imprints that you have been exposed to. Now we have some serious work to do because everyone needs inner child healing in our society. Trauma is a part of life: It exists in the world, and we are all exposed to it. Children internalize negative experiences, and it's these very experiences that will inevitably create the narrative for the child's inner landscape. When childhood is stable and loving, you learn to trust yourself and others, and that it is safe to embody and express your authentic truth. Your nervous system responds accordingly. Conversely, when childhood is unstable or traumatic, you learn that you cannot trust yourself, others, or your surroundings and again your nervous system responds and adapts accordingly. It primes you to exist in a state of hypervigilance and trains your mind to watch out for more traumatic experiences, inevitably setting you up to experience more of them.

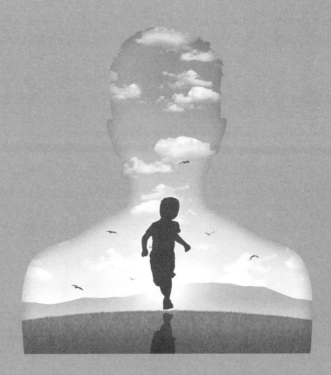

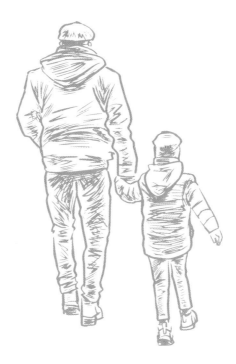

Working with the inner child allows you to heal deeper levels of your consciousness, where you can carefully learn to dismantle and escape these trauma loops. In this chapter, you will tap into your childlike nature, which will allow you to embody more creativity, playfulness, and joy. The creation of the shadow begins in childhood. It is essential to note that when we were children, most of us had to change our behaviors to match our parents' expectations. If we didn't behave to our parents' standards, most of us would receive some kind of scolding or punishment. Being punished, excluded, or ostracized as a child is a highly potent situation. We are wired to connect with others and to belong to a "tribe." Even though modern times have changed our lifestyles, we still have the same nervous systems as our ancestors. As humans, we evolved in close contact with our community, and so our fear of abandonment and rejection is more significant than our need for authenticity.

So, most of us keep hiding who we truly are and push parts of ourselves further into the unconscious, largely without even knowing it—thus creating a layered and abundant shadow. Certain behaviors and traits should be repressed, like murder, rape, violence, domination, abuse, or pedophilia. The problem occurs when innocent children are made to feel that normal behaviors belong in the shadow, such as questioning their parents' motives, rebelling against authority, acting out in anger or frustration, desiring to follow their own guidance systems, and making decisions based on how they feel. Strict parenting may produce a child who behaves politely, but it will create a massive shadow in its wake. I think we need to reformat parenting. First, it would be helpful if a lot more people had a general understanding of

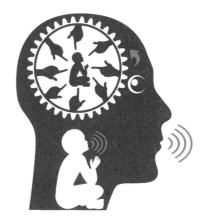

the shadow, the ego, and psychology in general. A parent who is comfortable with the existence of their own shadow aspects can help to hold space and support a child through their ego and shadow development. It is helpful to explain these concepts from an early age and to point them out when the child is showing shadow behavior, like lashing out in anger, hitting, taking things from others, not wanting to share or cooperate, and so on.

Pictures Are Worth a Thousand Words

Children's minds are like sponges; they pick up on so much of what's going on around them within their environment. But children usually do not have the language to properly verbalize what they are observing and experiencing. Nor do they have a mature frame of mind or adequate context from life experience to understand that negative scenarios aren't necessarily their fault, or their responsibility to fix. Children have a natural tendency to think the world revolves around them, which can unfortunately make abusive situations seem as though something is wrong with the child, rather than the abuser. All of this makes the process of being molded by our caretakers even more ingrained and impactful. As an adult, however, you can start to unpack and understand by putting words to your childhood memories and experiences, thereby giving you back a sense of control.

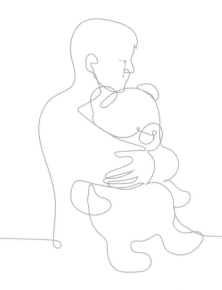

Looking Closer

One of the easiest ways to connect with your inner child is to remember yourself as a child. Go and find old pictures of yourself. Once you see yourself as a small, fragile child, you can really consider how innocent you were and begin to mourn the fact that you weren't allowed to be yourself exactly as you were. After all, a child doesn't understand the context behind their parents' negative statements; they only internalize them and think it's their own fault and that something must be wrong with them. Take time to grieve for the ways your authentic nature was stripped away from you.

Take Action

Find a few pictures of yourself as a child. Take time daily over the next week to connect with the photos and this childlike aspect of yourself. When practicing, try to put yourself into the mind frame of your inner child for five to ten minutes each day.

Below the Level of Consciousness

Babies and children utilize what are called mirror neurons to mimic their caretakers' behavior for learning social skills and language. In childhood, the brain wires the nervous system and the unconscious mind much like a hard drive. What is written is similar to the code in a computer system; it is challenging to override, especially from an awake or conscious state. As adults, editing this material is easily done from a relaxed, low-frequency brain wave state that is open to suggestion. It is essential to work with the shadow through altered states of consciousness to reach these transcendent brain wave frequencies.

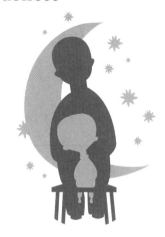

One crucial aspect of shadow work is to look at your childhood environment because that is the environment that shaped your consciousness. The shadow was formed along with the ego in response to what you experienced; it was a reaction, not an action in and of itself. It is not our fault that we have turned our back on ourselves—it was the price of admission into the family unit. Unpacking this with careful attention to detail will give you clues into your present and future when you begin to recognize the patterns at play.

Consider

••••◆◆◆◆◆◆••••

★ What are five keywords you would use to label your family's household growing up?
★ What are five keywords you would use to label your childhood in general?
★ What do these keywords reveal to you?
★ Is this what you would have expected, or are the words that you chose surprising in any way?

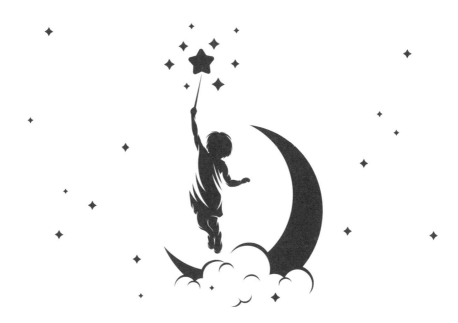

The Spark of Life

If you've ever spent any time with children, you will understand the innocence, curiosity, and pure joy that they emit. Children are born connected to their creativity, nature, and spirit. It's a shame the way this world breaks a young child's connection to these important resources and their own true nature. What happens to the spark that children have as they grow into adulthood? At first a bright flame, that spark is dimmed to a barely recognizable flicker. Instead of teaching children to be curious and to follow their intuition, we make up silly little curriculums and rules for them to follow, as if they aren't already infinitely intelligent just the way they are.

How often are you around children? They are such magical little creatures to watch: the way they let their curiosity guide their attention, the way their authentic little grins radiate pure joy and love. It's no wonder we must grind this abundant joy out of them before they can be expected to conform to society. It would be nice if children were at least allowed the span of their own childhood to just be a child, and not to worry about the weight of the world or the problems of their parents. However, for so many, this just isn't the case. It's time to dive deep into your childhood and the moments where your inner child suffered. Make a list of the times in your past when you felt like your inner child suffered. Explain each situation, then consider the following questions:

* How would you treat a child who felt like how you felt during those moments?
* If you were a small child (around one to seven years old), how would you take care of yourself if you were sad? Make a list of how you would talk to yourself and treat yourself with love and kindness.
* If you could treat yourself with more compassion every day, what would it look like?

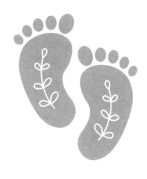

Treat Yourself

To a budding little human, bouncing off the walls with wonder and pure excitement, being forced to sit still must feel like torture. These are not the only wounds we face; we are also left to the programming of our parents, our family, the media, and society. Ever heard the phrase "Kids can be cruel"? Well, I'll let you in on a little secret: It's not the kids who are cruel. They are observing that behavior somewhere else. Children need so much love, so much energy, so much protection. They say our parents are our first teachers, which means many of us had teachers who expected their students to live up to their expectations—usually ones to validate themselves and their unfulfilled aspirations. Putting so much pressure on a child teaches them to put pressure on themselves. It teaches them to dismiss their own inner sensations of when to rest or when to act. This is great for keeping a prisoner under your control,

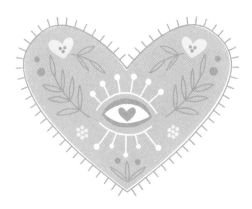

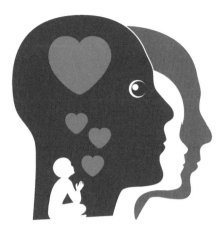

but it teaches children not to trust themselves. Once they grow up, this pattern tends to stick, as most patterns do.

Let compassion lead your inner child healing. This practice is so intuitive and so personal. We all have had different childhoods, and our healing will look different for each and every individual. However, the overarching theme for inner child work is compassion, always more compassion, because that is what we desperately need as children. In those moments when we were stripped of our innocence, we desperately needed an adult who had compassion for us—and for themselves, because how else could they cultivate it for us?

Take Action

- ★ Cultivate compassion and love for your inner child by treating yourself to something your childlike aspect would absolutely adore. Some examples are: taking an art class, spending time in nature, playing a game, or eating a special dish that reminds you of childhood.
- ★ What does your inner child need most from you? Take a moment to pause and ask them. Make a list in order of priority.
- ★ Set aside ten to fifteen minutes each day to give your inner child something from the list.

Take Your Power Back

Our inner children are indeed wounded. For most of us, we just buried them completely. We don't want to feel the wound of their existence even a little bit, because it's such a deep, gaping hole. I'm sure there are some exceptions to the rule; some children grow up in a "functional" household or one that is "good enough." But even those children were exposed to the larger outside world and everything that comes along with it, which almost always includes witnessing and experiencing a certain degree of trauma. I wonder what kind of world we could create with healed inner children. I'd like to think, generations far into the future, it would look like thriving and working together to bring about peace and harmony.

We can't go back and change the past (not literally anyway), but we do have the power to change our brain's feelings about the past by creating another outcome in place of the one that harmed us. The only power we have is over the present moment. From here we can clean up our past and therefore create a brighter future, not only for ourselves but for many generations to come. We break ancestral curses by healing one person at a time. We break down systems of oppression by collectively taking our power back from our oppressors—even when all that's left of them are remnants in our own minds.

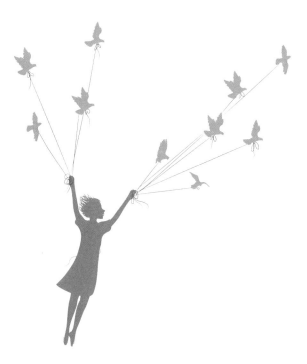

Since this powerlessness has been ingrained in us for so long, it can be hard to access it's root. Try this short exercise to dig deeper into your subconscious.

★ Think of a few situations where you felt like your power was stripped away from you as a child. Write them down in detail.
★ For each one, I want you to draw what that felt like. You can draw this however you feel called. Scribbles all over the page work; sometimes I've scribbled so hard I tear up the page a little bit. That's okay if it happens. Just try to draw whatever feels right.
★ Now I want you to draw an image of what it would look or feel like to take your power back in this situation. Again, maybe it's stick figures and scribbles or symbols and shapes. Whatever your subconscious mind wants, just draw, and don't judge what it looks like whatsoever.

Most people don't realize how profound the influence of our childhood really is. I suspect if it were more widely known, we would take extra precautions when raising our children. For many of us, childhood is a distant memory with some painful and sharp edges—sometimes with a few heartfelt and beautiful moments thrown in there as well. However, we must look at our inner child's wounds and explore more of our past in order to heal our present selves. Shadow work is making the sharp edges duller and finding the problem areas from our mental programming so that we may take the steering wheel of our consciousness back into our own hands. It's no longer necessary to play out the same stories that your ancestors did. You now have an awareness of the faulty programming and the power and the choice of whether or not you want to change it.

Take time to reexamine different areas of your life on a regular and consistent basis in order to keep integrating and actively seeking

Consider

When was the last time you played? For inner child healing, you must allow yourself more play in your life. Can you commit to more play? What would more play look like for you?

Take Action

Set aside ten to twenty minutes per day to play for ten days. This can be dancing, jumping on a trampoline, singing loudly in the shower or car, pressing every button on the elevator, playing ding–dong ditch . . . just don't hurt anyone or yourself.

individuation. If you wait long enough, all your shadow triggers will come up eventually, over and over again, until they are cleared of all their emotional charge through subconscious reprogramming. Healing is always cyclical; it also moves like a spiral. The same patterns come up again for deeper clearing in a perfect dance of awareness, practices of love and acceptance, and active integration. The closer you get to the center of the spiral, the more often the triggers show up for clearing. It's a perfect dance of universal truths expressing themselves through sentient beings: God watching God break down and heal infinitely.

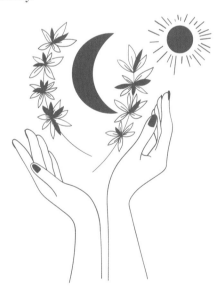

✳ ✳ ✳

6

TRAUMA AND THE IMPRINTS IT LEAVES BEHIND

Traumatic memories go deep into the unconscious mind for safekeeping because recalling a traumatic memory at the wrong moment can cause more psychological pain. Additionally, the mind protects you during the moment of trauma by shutting down into a state of altered consciousness—that way, you can navigate how to move forward in the moment without any hesitation or contemplation. We all have trauma; whether it comes from our upbringing or the outside world, we all need some form of healing. You must unpack your traumas to heal your core wounds—if you don't, you will not be able to see how they are leading you toward patterns of acting out unconsciously. Shadow work is finding out how we extract the antidote from the poison of pain. It is only during careful examination that we have this opportunity. Many traumas are hidden from us by our own brain, which is always trying to protect us. The brain can keep us stuck in trauma loops this way because it avoids thinking about or processing the very event that is continuously destabilizing it. Truly no one wants to hear this, but your trauma made you who you are. Your trauma was the chisel that shaped you from a formless block into a one-of-a-kind piece of art. Your trauma is the only thing that no one else can ever take away from you. It is unique to you, just like a fingerprint. That fingerprint alters you. It creates a new version of you after the traumatic experiences. The version of you before the trauma ceases to exist.

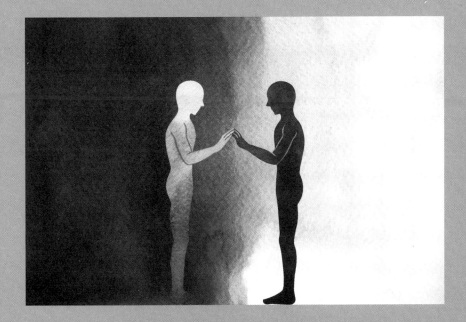

The trauma lives on inside the body, mind, and nervous system until it is processed. Sometimes this is a luxury we don't receive; many people are handed one trauma after another over their lifetime. Let's unpack the ways trauma affects people and how it was first discovered. We've known since the 1970s about PTSD and the effects of a singular, profound traumatic incident. We know that the brain and body do not know how to respond to extreme trauma or being scared to the point where death seems imminent. Most of what we first learned about PTSD was from studying Vietnam War veterans and the terrible nightmares, sensations, visions, and even hallucinations they came home with. A heroin epidemic surged right around this time. Many of the users were Vietnam vets desperately seeking some peace to quiet their inner turmoil, a way to sleep and rest their nervous systems that were still running on overdrive.

Traumatic Imprints

In *The Body Keeps the Score* (Penguin Books, 2014), trauma expert Bessel van der Kolk writes that people who have experienced trauma feel consistently unsafe. The frightening imprints of the past are alive within them in the form of chronic discomfort. Their innermost sensations are threatened with warning signs from the slightest shift in their environment. Since existing within the confines of the body is so incredibly painful, trauma victims learn to run from themselves.

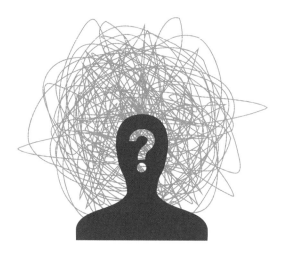

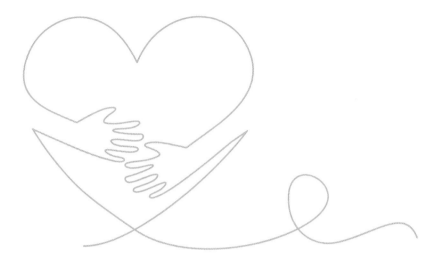

Trauma usually needs some kind of resolution within the mind of the experiencer in order to start a recovery process. This resolution comes from developing an understanding and compassion for the event and for the results created from it. This is indeed a complicated process, and sometimes frightening, but always worthwhile. For instance, how can one look at a car accident or a war crime with understanding and compassion? That is for each person to figure out by looking at the context of the situation and learning all the lessons one possibly can from the trauma.

Consider

⋯•◆◆◆◆◆•⋯

★ What are your five most impactful traumatic memories?
★ What did you feel in your body during each of these moments?
★ What is the core feeling left behind from each of the previous memories?
★ How have these memories shaped your internal narrative?
★ In what ways do you still protect yourself from this happening again?
★ Have you had this feeling or this situation come up again?

Trauma Changes the Brain

What changes in your brain once you've experienced trauma? Your stress response gets triggered by the nervous system: You are now in the fight, flight, freeze, or fawn mode (otherwise known as the "Four Fs of Trauma Response"). When the limbic system, the part of the brain that plays a role in behavioral and emotional responses, is activated by trauma, your thought process basically reverts to a more primal state, where your only job is to judge your immediate circumstances for safety or threat. At this point, your brain does not prioritize rational thinking. A resolution is needed so your priorities can get back in order. Sometimes the resolution is just resting or sharing the experience.

So, what happens when our wires get crossed from history with an abusive caretaker, and we are constantly feeling threatened, even by safe situations? Our nervous system is working overtime, always keeping us on guard in case of a potential threat—creating a hypervigilant state where one's body begins to show signs of "dis-ease" after enough time. We must fully dissect our previous traumas to process and integrate what is needed and come to a resolution. Reprogramming is necessary to discharge the trauma in the mind, body, and nervous system.

The Brain's Response to Trauma			
Amygdala	Hypothalamus	Hippocampus	Prefrontal Cortex
The Alarm Center	The Operations Manager	The Biographer	The CEO
Detects threats	Releases stress hormones	Retrieves memories from the past	Analyzes information and designs a response
Starts stress response	Prepares you for fight or flight	Anticipates what will happen	Creates a plan to respond to stress

Consider

······◆◆◆◆◆◆······

* ★ In what ways have the traumas you detailed previously changed you into a new version of yourself?
* ★ Are there any lessons that you learned or still need to learn from each event?
* ★ What do you wish happened instead? Create a resolution in your mind.
* ★ Take a few minutes before bed each night and envision what you wish would have happened instead of what did, thereby reprogramming your subconscious and creating a resolution for your mind.

Complex Trauma

It wasn't until the year 1988 that complex PTSD (CPTSD) was discovered. It develops from long-term traumas, sometimes less explicit but with the potential to be infinitely more insidious. CPTSD frequently develops in childhood, with parents wracked with addiction, narcissism, self-loathing, or mental health disorders like severe depression. These emotional scars take years to develop, and they can create an unstable foundation for the child's internal narrative and self-concept when they grow up with prolonged neglect or abuse, whether it is emotional in nature or exacerbated by violence.

CPTSD can develop due to emotional abuse; sometimes the abuse is subtle and not evident to the abused person until looked at through another lens, usually during shadow work or therapy. I would bet many chronic illness and mental health patients are sufferers of CPTSD, PTSD, and unresolved trauma—their symptoms arising because mental turmoil and hypervigilance were thought to be their normal state, and therefore not deemed unusual in their experience.

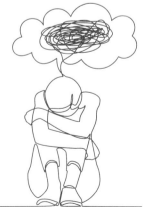

Changing Your Emotional State

I want you to unpack the feelings you generate when you recall childhood memories. This feeling is tied to an emotional state. The more you can proactively work to change your emotional state when you feel weighed down with negativity, depression, feeling stuck, or low energy, the more control you will have over your consciousness and your life. You will also find it much easier to accomplish goals.

* What are the feelings you experience when you remember childhood memories?
* Have you ever made a correlation between your mental state and your physical state? Starting now, the next time you're feeling off, write about what thoughts and feelings preceded it.
* What thoughts, feelings, and actions make you feel like you are in a good emotional state?
* What are some tools you can use when you feel like your mental state is off? (For example, dancing, taking a walk, exercising, cooking, taking a bath, getting some sunlight, journaling, etc.)
* How can you cultivate more awareness of what state you are in each moment and take action to change it when you need to?

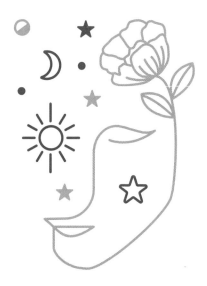

Restorative Yoga for Healing Trauma

While a person who experiences one impactful trauma could potentially rebound very well with the right support directly after the event, a CPTSD survivor has much more work to do to make the world feel safe. The degree of safety we feel in any given moment is a key indicator to our body and brain as to whether we need to be hypervigilant to protect ourselves, or we can relax. Often for a CPTSD survivor, safety is not an accessible feeling until much of their trauma work is processed.

It takes ongoing work to rebalance the nervous system, especially if you have PTSD or CPTSD. Let's try some supportive and restorative yoga poses that will gently allow your body to come into a deeper sense of relaxation and a deeper connection with yourself. You can do these in any order and hold them for as long as you feel comfortable.

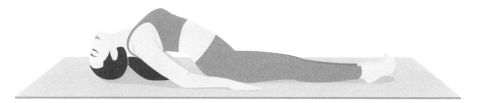

Fish Pose (Matsyasana)

Lie down, letting your legs and arms sprawl out comfortably to the sides, with palms facing up. Press your head to the mat and arch your upper back, using your arms to help press your shoulders down. Breathe deeply and stay as long as you desire.

> **Benefits:** This is a gentle restorative backbend. The goal is to relax and to open the front body. Trauma causes poor posture due to body armoring. This will simultaneously help with posture and with restoring the nervous system.

★ After doing this pose, did you notice that you're sitting up or walking a bit straighter?

★ Take stock of your mental energy after holding this pose. Does your mind feel less cluttered?

★ Did you notice a physical release in your spine?

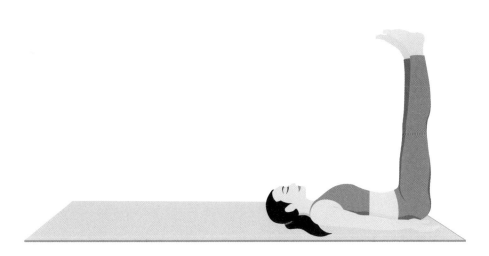

Legs Up the Wall (Viparita Karani)

This one is so easy you can do it almost anywhere. Find a place where you can rest with your legs against a wall. Sit down on the floor and scoot your butt as close to the wall as possible. Then swing your legs up the wall slowly and gently, while lying down—either with your back flat on the ground or with a blanket or bolster. Relax here with long, deep breaths for about five to ten minutes.

> **Benefits:** Having your legs higher than your head and your heart is known as an inversion. It can reduce blood pressure and reduce blood pooling in some parts of the body temporarily, which helps to refresh circulation throughout your body. If you are stressed, fatigued, or feeling triggered, this pose is especially relaxing and perfect for stress relief.

★ After doing this pose, did you notice a change in your heart rate or breathing?

★ As your circulation improves, how is that impacting your emotional state?

★ In what ways can you incorporate this pose into your daily life?

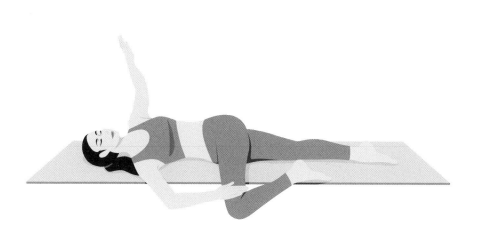

Reclined Twist (Supta Matsyendrasana)

Lie down on your back and hug your knees into your torso. Open your arms outward in a T shape on the floor, relaxing your shoulders to the ground. One at a time, bring your knee down to rest on the floor across your body, using your hand to press it gently to the ground. Stay for a few minutes and repeat on the other side.

> **Benefits:** A twisting pose helps to compress the internal organs, easing the digestive system. It can also help to relieve stress. Twisting helps to restore equilibrium in the nervous system and releases tension in the spine.

★ After doing this pose on each side, do you feel a sense of safety?

★ Notice your gut and spine. What physical improvements are you feeling?

★ What about your state of mind? As the blood flow nourishes your body, do you find that it also improves your outlook?

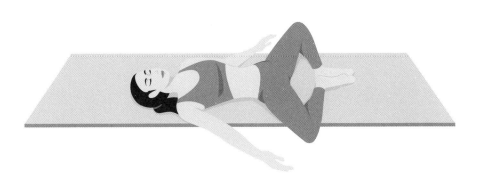

Reclined Butterfly (Supta Baddha Konasana)

Gently lie down on your yoga mat. If you like, you can place a blanket or a cushion underneath your head. Bring the soles of your feet together and pull them up toward your hips. Let your knees bend out to the sides. Add cushions or a yoga block under each thigh for added support, if desired. I like to put one hand on my heart and one on my belly in this pose, but they can also rest gently beside you.

> **Benefits:** This pose helps to improve blood circulation and stretches the inner thigh and groin areas. It helps to relieve symptoms of stress, anxiety, and depression.

★ After holding this pose for several minutes, take inventory of your stress level. Do you feel a shift in your anxiety?

★ With circulation improved, do you feel a connection between your mind and body?

★ When do you feel you need to do this pose the most?

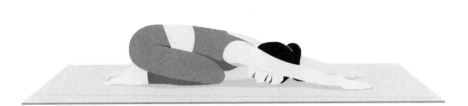

Child's Pose (Bālāsana)

If you choose, grab a bolster or a few blankets folded into a rectangle and place it between the legs before lying down. Sit on your heels, with your knees spread wider than your hips. Then, slowly and gently fold down until your belly is comfortably resting between your legs (or on the bolster and blankets if you choose to use them) and your forehead is on the mat or a pillow. Extend the arms straight out in front of you for a deeper stretch or leave them resting alongside the body.

> **Benefits:** This is a healing, restorative pose that gently stretches the spine. They call it "child's pose" because it is very psychologically soothing when you're feeling triggered, anxious, or vulnerable.

★ When you encounter a stressful situation, how can you take a few solitary moments to relax and recenter yourself by doing child's pose?

★ When you come out of the pose, notice your heart center. Does it still feel tight and anxious, or are you feeling a release of anxiety?

★ While in this pose, are you able to focus on just the present moment?

The Four Fs of Trauma Response

There are four common ways people respond to trauma. These responses are called the four Fs: Fight, Flight, Freeze, and Fawn. *Fight* is when your reaction to a stress response is to fight against the threat because you think you can overpower it. *Flight* is when your reaction is a decision to run away from the perceived danger, which may very well be your best option in some cases. *Freeze* is when you feel stuck and you are not able to act—think of a deer in the headlights. The *fawn* response is typical of children who grew up in abusive families, and who had to adapt to please the abuser in order to survive.

Overuse of these trauma responses creates problems for the survivor after the responses are adapted for a length of time. For instance, people who favor the flight response to trauma may have extremely high cortisol levels and burned-out adrenals; they are frequently workaholics who escape pain through busyness. Another example is those who favor the fight response: They often act narcissistic and use control to bully others to distract them from their own pain. A freeze response type can leave a person stuck in a depressed state, hardly able to do anything at all. And those who favor the fawn response become the ultimate people pleasers, ignoring any needs they have for themselves.

I think it's crucial we all learn about trauma and how its impacts don't cease once the event is over. The brain and the body will always remember the trauma it's been through. This is not to hurt you but to try to keep you safe from another traumatic incident. With ongoing shadow work, you can develop compassion for yourself and your nervous system and continue to seek out lessons from your discomfort—both in the past and into the future.

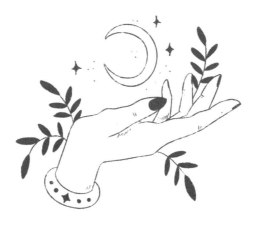

Take Action

In your journal, write your answers to the following questions. If you find that these are difficult to ponder, try stopping intermittently and doing your favorite yoga pose from earlier in the chapter. What are the trauma responses that you recognize you use the most? In what ways does this affect your life? How do you know when you're in a trauma response? What tools work best for you to come out of your trauma response? In what ways have your trauma responses become a part of your personality?

As you continue through this book and with shadow work, you will likely gain access to deeper levels of your subconscious and unconscious mind. You may also gain access to traumatic memories you had previously blocked out. I encourage you to take this as a sign you are accessing deeper levels of your consciousness and therefore deeper levels of healing. If at any time you feel like the information coming to the surface is too big of a burden to bear, please seek additional support, such as a therapist.

Come back to the following questions as deeper things come to the surface for you during your shadow work:

★ What memories had I intentionally blocked out?
★ How do I feel now that I have access again? Am I ready to heal this memory by subconscious reprogramming?
★ What do I wish happened instead of what actually happened? Take time and visualize the desired outcome instead of the real one. Repeat as much as possible.

7

CALM THE NERVOUS SYSTEM, COME HOME TO THE BODY

The current way in which the world operates is extremely taxing to your nervous system. Learning to calm down and deeply relax will benefit you in more ways than you know. After learning about your nervous system in this chapter, you will understand that you may have been deeply impacted by your traumatic experiences thus far. The fact is, it is challenging to work on self-improvement when you are already feeling on edge. To access deeper levels of healing, you must make rest a priority. You will learn about and explore ways to relax and be grounded after all the important shadow work you've been processing so far. You'll explore practices that will allow your body to discern information in order to set healthy boundaries. We need to build trust again and learn to embody our own sacredness without holding back due to our unconscious wounds. So often, people who have experienced trauma live in an out-of-body experience. We must learn to come home to the body and continue to exist within the boundaries of our skin. The body is our home; let us come back to it.

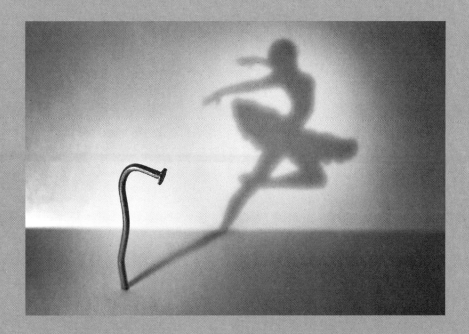

The human brain and nervous system have developed over the span of two million years. It has saved our ancestors from predators and enemies alike. During most of that time frame, we lived very different lives compared to our modern lifestyles. In the past, we had to outrun our food, hunt and kill to eat, and work long hours gathering sustenance just to survive. For a great deal of that time, we lived without shelter, with constant threats looming in the darkness. It's so imperative that people begin to learn about their own nervous systems and how we are all affected by trauma, both in our own lives and systemically on a larger scale. Chronic fight-or-flight responses will cause a person to distract themselves from inner turmoil. We need practices that remind our nervous system to rest and relax so we may digest our food properly and sleep well because this helps to prevent disease. In this chapter, I will share nervous system hacks with you so you will have tools when you realize you are stuck in a stress response.

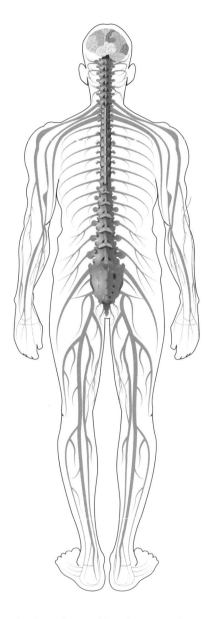

Using shadow work, you will begin to look at the world and the people in it very differently. You will gain so much understanding just by making a rapid assessment of their internal workings. Because, when you know how to look for them, they are all displayed outwardly in one way or another.

Box Breath

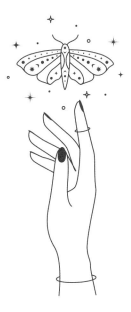

The four-F responses were developed so that we would have an opportunity to escape from danger. When the limbic system is triggered, our brains effectively prioritize an emotional response over rational thinking. During a stress response, your mental energy is redirected to your limbic system, meaning you may not always react rationally to stressful moments or perceived threats.

Because shadow work will inevitably have some destabilizing moments, we will work with some basic tools to help you rebalance your nervous system. This exercise will use the breath. This is a simple and easy-to-remember exercise—if it works for you. Breathwork doesn't work for a lot of trauma survivors because if you are still working through trauma, it feels so scary to be in the body and aware of your breath. If this exercise makes you feel uncomfortable, don't do it. You don't have to force it.

Let's try a box breathing technique to calm anxiety and help restore the nervous system back to balance:

★ Start by breathing in slowly through your nose while counting to five. Feel the air fill up your lungs.

★ Hold the breath for five seconds. Exhale slowly out of your mouth for five seconds and hold for another five seconds. Repeat for eleven minutes.

★ Practice three times per week.

★ Each time you practice, write down what thoughts come up for you during this exercise.

★ After practicing for one month, come back to your notes. What patterns do you notice in your thoughts?

Rewiring the Fear Response

The amygdala is the region of the brain that is activated during moments of stress, and it controls your fear and anger responses. The amygdala sends signals to the hypothalamus, which stimulates the autonomic nervous system to release cortisol and adrenaline, aka stress hormones. Too much cortisol and adrenaline in your body can be very damaging to it. Here are some simple nervous system hacks for you to try out. These should help you come out of your fear response and back to nervous system balance. Try them all and figure out which ones work best for you.

- ★ **Physical activity**—Doing something physical enough to stimulate your body (but not enough to stress you out) is the fastest and easiest way to come out of a stress response. Think of dancing, yoga, stretching, taking a walk, qigong, etc.
- ★ **Touch**—Another fast and easy way to get out of a stress response is to give someone a hug for twenty seconds. Our nervous system recognizes this from many lifetimes of our ancestors coming home from the dangers of the outside world to a warm, welcoming embrace from their loved ones. Touch stimulates oxytocin, the love hormone, which has been proven to decrease stress.

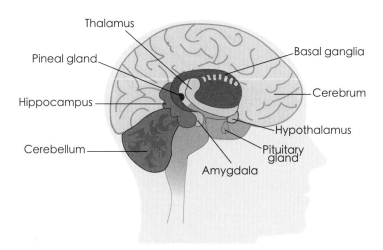

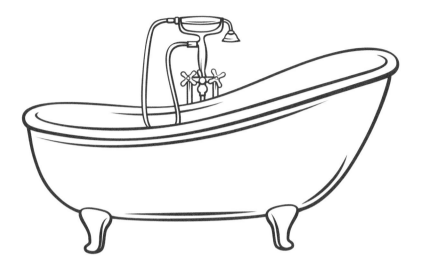

★ **Shake it off**—Shaking your body (like we've all seen a dog do after a bath) activates the parasympathetic nervous system and tells the brain to relax and let go. Shaking will also stimulate the lymphatic system, which helps our body with detoxing.

★ **Warmth** (hot bath, warm sun, heating pad)—I think we've all felt better after a relaxing bath at one time or another. Hot baths also help to reduce inflammation.

★ **Turn down the volume**—By reducing unnecessary stimuli like bright lights, loud noises, or constant background noise, we can help to send a message to the nervous system that we are in a safe environment. This will help stimulate the parasympathetic nervous system and take you out of a stress response.

★ **Eat more healthy fats**—Nerve cells are wrapped in a protective coating called myelin, which is an insulating layer that forms around nerves like the ones in the brain and spine. Myelin is made of protein and fatty substances. This protective sheath allows nerve cells to transmit electrical impulses quickly and efficiently. If your myelin is damaged, these impulses will slow down. Eating fats can help keep this protective coating healthy; fats are a way to literally cushion your nervous system. An easy way to eat healthy fats is to follow a Mediterranean diet rich in seafood, olive oil, nuts, and seeds.

Somatic Experiencing

When we experience trauma in childhood or over an extended length of time, our four-F response becomes easily triggered, and it becomes more difficult to turn it off. Small things, such as a negative comment on your social media, may trigger you into a full-blown fight, flight, freeze, or fawn response. It may take hours or even days for you to calm your nervous system and come back to equilibrium—and that's if you know you are triggered and are actively trying to restore balance.

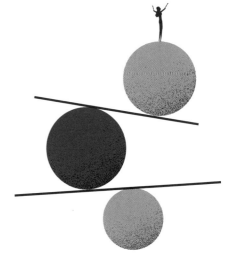

Many people who experience trauma don't realize when they are in fact in a trauma response, and they don't have a chance to regain a sense of control over their mind and body before it gets triggered all over again. Unfortunately, some people experience trauma so frequently that they rarely have a moment in their bodies without this stress response turned on. That's why it's so crucial to learn to notice when you are triggered and utilize some of these practical tools to bring you back to equilibrium.

Take Action

Tracking is a somatic experiencing technique that will help you feel grounded. Take a few breaths and focus your energy on feeling relaxed. When you feel ready, begin to look around the room and notice different objects. As you observe, name the object out loud if you are alone or in your mind if you are not alone. If you find something that holds your attention, stay with it. Keep finding new objects until you feel a sense of calm.

Resourcing

I want you to try a simple tool called resourcing. It's a somatic experiencing tool to help you access a sense of peace. Here's how it works: When you feel a nervous system response or trigger, you will work on bringing positive memories of a place, person, or something you love to the forefront of your mind. Resourcing can help you stay calm as you experience trauma sensations and/or memories of the event. Next time you feel triggered, I want you to try this resourcing tool.

Consider

★ What is it that triggered you?
★ What positive memory did you bring to the forefront of your mind?
★ How did your nervous system feel?
★ Do you feel like this tool worked well for you? Why or why not?
★ Would you use this tool again?

Parasympathetic Nervous System Activators

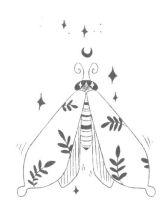

Trauma alters who we are in a profound way. In *The Body Keeps the Score*, Bessel van der Kolk explains that experiences that overwhelm our nervous system change our inner sensations and our relationship to our physical reality. Trauma, therefore, is not just an event that took place in the past but a very real imprint left within the consciousness, brain, and body that can affect us indefinitely. The book goes on to talk about how, after traumatic experiences, a reorganization takes place in the way the mind and body manage perceptions. Not only does trauma change the way that we think, but it also actually changes our capacity *to* think, and even what we think about.

When our fear center is activated, we are flooded with stress hormones and bodily sensations to accompany them, such as a racing heart, shallow breath, tightness in the chest, or numbness in the legs. In one study, trauma patients undergoing MRIs were shown images that reminded them of their traumatic experiences. Their scans showed a huge decrease in blood flow to the frontal cortex of the brain, resembling images of stroke patients. Let's explore some more nervous system exercises or hacks to bring us out of sympathetic dominance and back to parasympathetic rest and digest mode.

Sitali Breath

Roll your tongue, letting it stick out of your mouth slightly. Inhale for four seconds, bringing your tongue in at the end, then exhale through the nose for six seconds. This will feel challenging in the beginning, but it will get easier. This breath creates pressure in your lungs that helps to regulate your nervous system; the longer exhale tells your nervous system that you are safe.

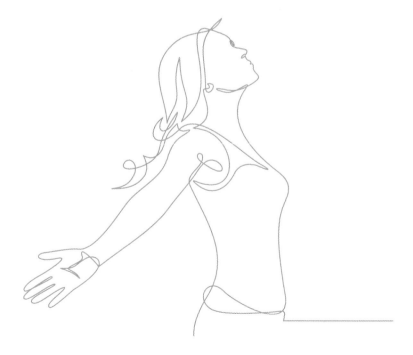

Bilateral Stimulation

Stimulating both sides of the brain at the same time redirects intense energy. During a four-F response, we have excess energy, with brain waves concentrating in the amygdala. It's easy to activate both sides of the brain by grabbing an object and passing it from one hand to the other while your eyes follow.

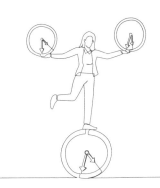

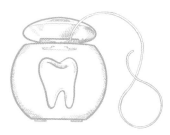

Flossing

While you floss, you drop your jaw, which is a way of signaling to your body that all is okay, therefore reducing stress. When you're getting ready to fight, you will naturally brace your jaw, which triggers a fight-or-flight response. When we drop the jaw, we're telling our nervous system we are safe.

Hug Yourself

Cross your arms in front of your chest and put one hand on each shoulder. Apply gentle pressure on your skin as you slowly slide your hands down your arms. In your upper body, there are nerve endings right underneath the surface of your skin. When you apply gentle pressure to these nerve endings, it creates delta waves in your brain.

Vagus Nerve Stimulation

For true healing to take place, we need to remind the body that the danger has since passed. We also need to be able to live in the present reality where one can find some inner peace. This is difficult because whenever the trauma experiencer witnesses any sensory input that reminds the nervous system of the trauma, the limbic system and the amygdala are immediately triggered. This sends the person into a four-F response, most of the time before they even realize it.

This cranial nerve communicates with the parasympathetic system's control of the digestive tract, lungs, and heart. The word *vagus* in Latin means "wandering." They named this cranial nerve vagus because it is the longest cranial nerve; it travels from the brainstem all the way to part of the colon. When stimulated, this nerve can help bring you back to a balanced state by turning off your stress response. Try some activities such as mild exercise, getting a massage, gargling water, or initiating a positive social interaction. A cold shower or splashing cool water on your face is a good way to reset; you can also spend time in nature or speak softly and rhythmically as if you were soothing a child.

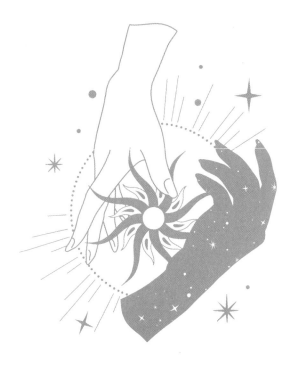

Take Action

When you feel that other actions aren't working to calm you, use the Valsalva Maneuver. Try to exhale, but keep your mouth closed and pinch your nose like you're trying to clear your ear pressure on a plane. This increases the pressure inside your chest cavity, which stimulates your vagus nerve.

We live in a world with many stressors that essentially promote sympathetic dominance in most people. However, we also have science and human biohacking technology to rewire ourselves to feel safe regardless. Our brain is in constant survival mode; it is always working hard to protect us, and it does the best job possible. That is why you are here, still alive 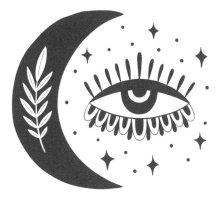 and reading this book. We must apply these techniques the moment we notice our stress response is turned on. Find what works for you. Try all of the tools a few times; they won't always work for certain stressors, which is why it is essential to have different ones within your toolbox.

I want you to create a shortcut list for when you get triggered in daily life. This way you'll have tools to accompany you during your stress response that will hopefully bring you back to equilibrium quickly and efficiently. If, however, you only use these tools to try them out and then forget to draw upon them when triggered, you'll be doing yourself a disservice that will prolong unnecessary stress.

❋   ❋   ❋

8

TRIGGERS ARE TEACHERS, PEOPLE ARE MIRRORS

One of the shadow's only ways to communicate with your conscious awareness is to cause an emotional reaction to a trigger. Every time you are triggered, the shadow is pointing to an area within you that still needs healing. After a nervous system reaction to a trigger has passed, you can look at triggers like a treasure chest revealing where your deepest integration is available. Once you learn to handle triggers effectively from this book, you can use them as clues to guide you in healing the portion of your shadow that is crying out for attention. You've learned practices to help you cope with triggers by grounding and utilizing your body. Now you can influence your mind to relax under stress and avoid acting out unconsciously. You will learn to write down triggers to discover more information after the intense emotional reaction has passed. That is how you will know where hidden psychological pain exists in your shadow. With more investigation, you can determine where the trigger stems from, allowing healing on a deeper level. You will also learn about projection, a powerful tool the shadow uses to shed light on where our weak points are.

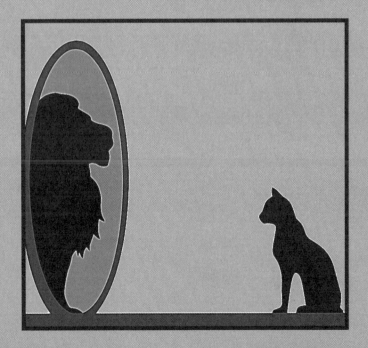

People Are Mirrors

Have you ever heard the phrase "Other people are your mirror"? I'm not sure if the person who first used this phrase knew how true this actually is. I know that I heard this concept a few times before I ever found out about shadow work, but I guess I just let it go in one ear and out the other, because I never really paid any attention to it, or even bothered to contemplate what it meant. Now I'm deeply aware of this powerful phrase. It serves as a compass to steer me back to myself when I find I'm wanting to place blame for my emotions outward or compare myself to others. This doesn't take into account that we experience trauma that we most certainly did not deserve, such as neglect or abuse in childhood (or even as an adult)—obviously having done nothing to create it. Some folks believe this can be karmic retribution for wrongdoings from past lives. I won't delve into that topic in this book, but it's interesting to consider. I'll admit, though, that it's not very helpful or empowering.

You're probably wondering what I mean when I partially named this chapter "Triggers Are Teachers." What I mean is, the shadow has very few tools to use to gain your attention. A trigger is one of those tools, which it uses because it desperately craves integration, acknowledgment, and balance. So, when we are triggered, we must explore what that trigger is bringing up. In other words: What core wound is this trigger pointing to? I know it's not always easy to explore this kind of thing when we are in a nervous system response. I always recommend using nervous system tools (which we went over in chapter seven) and then waiting until you feel calm, cool, and collected before trying to explore your trigger further.

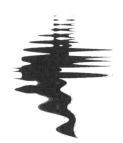

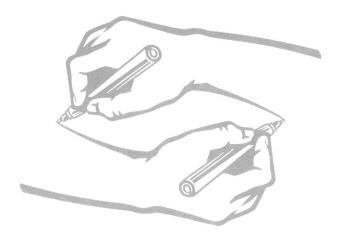

The World Is Your Mirror

Triggers are created by the mind to protect us from experiencing psychological pain because the mind avoids pain at all costs. Earlier in this book, you learned that as we grow into adulthood, we develop ourselves around avoiding pain. However, when pain is present and unavoidable, such as with a toxic caregiver, we develop unhealthy coping mechanisms like people pleasing.

These coping mechanisms allow us to survive the abuse, but they are damaging in the long run. We begin to develop an unhealthy, false personality around the constant stress-response triggers. Once you can cognitively recognize that triggers are actually pointing out pieces of you that still need healing, then you realize they are your teachers. And if you are on a journey of healing, they are like breadcrumbs leading you through uncharted territory.

Consider

If the world is a mirror, what is it showing you right now? Draw an image that your subconscious brings up for you, then take some time to translate what it means to you. How do you feel about your life? About your circumstances? Your future? Your work? Your friends?

Shining a Light on Envy

Let's talk about projection. Who do you resent, envy, or hate? When you are pointing a finger in blame at another person, notice you still have three fingers pointed back at you. You know that idol you've put on a pedestal? That is an example of where you are afraid to take up space and be seen; it is your golden shadow. That person you detest and can't stop complaining about? Something in them is triggering a shadow within you, and it's up to you to figure out exactly what needs healing.

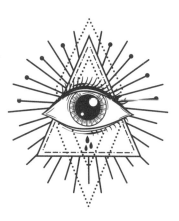

Your Protective Brain

Envy and resentment are just more tools the mind uses to protect you. Instead of creating an uncomfortable realization about something within your shadow, the mind uses projection instead, convincing you that someone else deserves your animosity. This serves as a distraction, a safer way for the mind to process feelings without attaching them to us because the ego would absolutely hate that. Try this: In your journal, make a list of the people you admire or envy. Write down the qualities or attributes that make you envy them. Pick something from the list and visualize what you would look like if you had this quality and how that makes you feel. Make a list of all the ways that embodying this quality would change your life. Think about how your life would transform if you had this. If you end up deciding it would be beneficial, work on embodying this by stepping out of your comfort zone as if you already possess it.

Put Yourself in Their Shoes

It's important to notice when your thoughts are completely preoccupied with someone else. Projection feels more intense than being irritated or annoyed, the main difference being an inability to take your focus off the other person or group of people. Blaming and self-justification feel like an endless spiral. Turn inward to help heal the projection—because, by definition, projection is focusing outward. Shift into self-awareness mode and begin to notice how you feel. How is

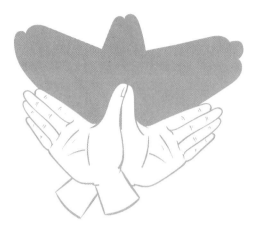

your breath? Are you tensing your muscles? The awareness of your own bodily sensations should help to break the cycle of obsessive thoughts about the person who is harboring your projection.

Looking Closer

One of the easiest ways we can end a cycle of projection is to do our best to put ourselves in the other person's shoes and to diligently try to look at things from their viewpoint for a moment. This will give you a whole new perspective. Use the following writing prompts to do just that:

* ★ Write about the irritating person or situation using third-person language (he, she, or it). You have full permission to let it all out.
* ★ Now write about the same irritating person or situation as if you were having a conversation with them. Tell them what's been bothering you and listen to their responses, whatever they might be. Use your imagination and respond with the first thing that comes to mind.
* ★ Next, write from this person's point of view using first-person language, referring to yourself in the third person. Write down what you think they would think and say about you after the previous prompt. This may feel uncomfortable but do your best to be honest with yourself. This is all about you and changing your perspective.
* ★ Last, review what you wrote so far and ponder what it all means. What do you suspect is the real underlying issue? What made you feel that way?

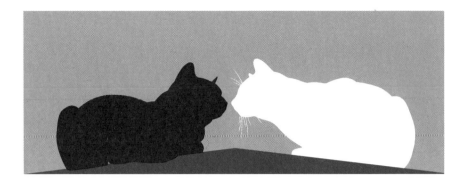

Current Issues on the Horizon

Once you understand how everyone serves as a mirror for your own internal self-conflict, you will gain so much power and awareness over the ways your mind leaks invaluable energy. It's crucial to achieving your goals and fulfilling your desires. If you want to harness every ounce of your will toward a deeper, more meaningful life, and fulfill your authentic purpose, you can't be using your energy in this unconscious way any longer.

Projection is a tool we use to try to protect ourselves in many different ways. When we're hurt or rejected, we blame the other person, our circumstances, or even ourselves, because having something to blame feels like a resolution to our mind. Blaming feels like a relief, but it ignores the deeper issue, which is discovering what the discomfort is pointing to.

Take Action

Take notice of any issues that arise in daily life over the next five days. Create a journal entry for each one and explain the situation. After five days, come back and review. Do you notice some recurring issues coming up in your life? What patterns do you see? If you don't see any patterns yet, keep this question in your mind for the next few days and continue to take notes on issues that come up for you. Journal anything that comes to mind. Do you remember anything from your past that reminds you of this pattern in any way?

Explosive Triggers

Our minds work in overdrive to keep us from feeling uncomfortable feelings. Our emotions are all so jumbled up that we don't even allow ourselves the space to experience them. Most people couldn't tell you what anger actually feels like in their body—the somatic, physical symptoms that accompany it, such as a racing heart, tightness in the chest, hot skin, feeling numb, etc. Anger is such a misunderstood emotion. Did you know it is a secondary emotion? It actually stems from fear or sadness.

Anxiety and worry trigger fear. Loss and disappointment trigger sadness. Feeling these intense emotions is uncomfortable. They provoke vulnerability, which can make a person feel like they are losing control. That's usually when people unconsciously decide to feel anger instead, in order to avoid the discomfort of vulnerability that comes with fear or sadness. Anger gives a person a surge of energy and usually something to blame and direct their anger at, which gives the illusion of control.

The process of allowing the discomfort when you experience triggers is not easy, but it's incredibly valuable, and it takes your power back from the situation. It's cathartic once you have begun to master it. People you label "difficult" possess some of the same negative traits you disown in yourself.

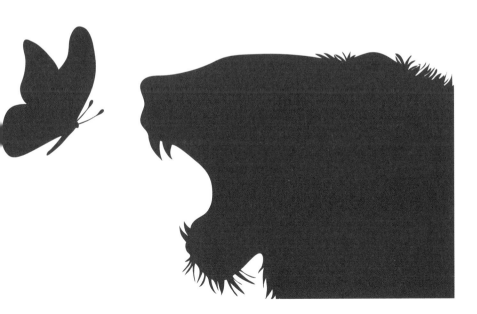

Consider

* What are the three biggest triggers you can remember? What did it make you feel like, and what was the result?
* Now, what was your part? (We all have a part, even if it was just "I was there." It doesn't mean you are to blame for what happened.)
* What is the shadow trying to show you through another person? Is this a pattern? Who else have you had a similar experience with?
* What feelings is your shadow asking you to lean into? What steps can you take to lean into these feelings?

We usually find a person who fits the behavior we are trying to project. This means you will project bullying onto a person who is actually a bully—but you are projecting due to disowning this behavior within yourself. You may be avoiding admitting to yourself that you can sometimes be a bit of a bully as well. Or maybe you weren't allowed to stick up for yourself at all, and you're triggered because you had to put standing up for yourself into your shadow.

Try to look at the other person in their full humanity. Take their negative behavior in the right context and realize they have positive qualities as well. Alternatively, if they are truly toxic, you must create boundaries to shield yourself and to stop using them as a screen on which you project your own disowned aspects. Trade places with the other person. Ask yourself, "How would I feel if I knew somebody was thinking about me the way I'm thinking about _____?" This can help transform the other person from a symbol of what you don't like (in yourself) into a human being—who, like you, is probably just doing the best they can.

Copy the following list and place it somewhere you have easy access to so that you can refer to it when you're feeling triggered. Which practices work best for you?

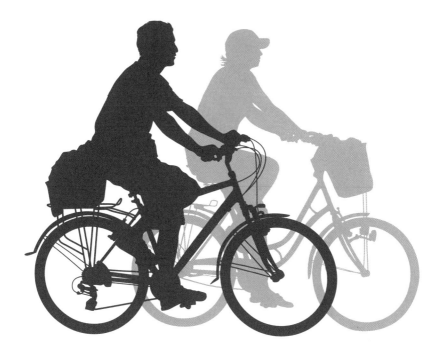

★ Slow, conscious breathing
★ A cold shower or splashing cold water on your face
★ Mild exercise, like riding a bike
★ Getting a massage
★ Gargling
★ Positive social interactions
★ Humming, singing, or chanting
★ Valsalva Maneuver
★ Speaking softly and rhythmically
★ Spending time in nature

9

CONTINUE THE HEALING JOURNEY

A daily inventory will help you as you move forward with shadow work beyond this book. Now that you have successfully confronted hidden aspects of yourself—including your ego, shadow, and inner child, all guided by your higher self—you now have all the tools necessary to become the steward of your consciousness in any way that you desire. However, this will require consistency on your part. We will always have more shadow to be illuminated, and you want to refrain from adding more unconscious energy to it. That is what this chapter is for. I will provide you with a simple daily inventory to go through each night to make sure you go to bed with total awareness. I will also provide you with a weekly, monthly, and yearly check-in, as well as an inventory for when you are triggered, resentful, or envious, and one for when you're feeling disconnected. This way you will be able to go over things with a fine-tooth comb, thus helping you become aware of your patterns and change them. Shadow work helps to dissolve limiting beliefs and negative programming, so it's crucial to keep it consistent. It takes time to reprogram the subconscious mind because it uses repetition to rewrite faulty programming.

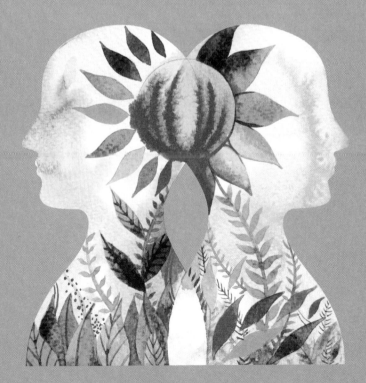

Have you ever been to the beach and written your name in the sand by the water? You may remember the waves washing those letters away, little by little, until they've faded back into plain sand. When you rewire your subconscious mind, I want you to think of this image. The old memory will slowly vanish the more often you do it, as each wave washes away the letters a little more each time. You are then actively writing something new over the old again and again, eventually canceling out the other programming or memory. The point

of this analogy is it takes time to rewrite and dissolve information in the subconscious. It is not instantaneous. An inventory allows you to catch issues and problems before they arise in your life. It will allow you to go to bed with a clear conscience, or at least an idea of how to gain one. It will keep you from holding resentments and grudges. It will help you uphold your boundaries and remind you to take care of yourself. An inventory will show you your patterns in real time, so you can heal those that work against you. It will help you cultivate awareness and take personal responsibility for your thoughts, feelings, and actions.

Daily Inventory

To reap the abundant benefits available, shadow work is a process that you should continue to practice over the course of a lifetime. The more you can confront the shadow and your own consciousness, the more you will feel grounded, content, and gracefully detached from the outcome. As I like to say: Confront the shadow, get the gold. A daily inventory will make the process simple and easy. This practice will be very revealing if you keep it up.

Take Action

••••◆◆◆◆◆◆••••

Take a moment to check in with yourself and write down any clues that the shadow may be trying to reveal to you. Afterward, ask yourself the following questions. If you feel compelled, you can write your answers in your journal. You don't need to write very much if you don't feel called— just a few words or a sentence is enough. Stay consistent for thirty days and see how much of a difference it makes!

Before you go to bed at the end of each day, take a few moments to answer the following questions:

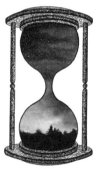

- ★ What has occurred throughout your day that was aggravating or upsetting?
- ★ Where could you have had more awareness?
- ★ How did you take care of your body?
- ★ How did you take care of your mental health?
- ★ How did you uphold your boundaries?
- ★ Did your shadow show up today? If so, how?

Weekly Inventory

A lot can happen in a week. If you don't take time to slow down and look back at what happened, it might just pass you by. We are all learning lessons every single day, important life lessons that are so priceless and valuable that we should take time to acknowledge them and congratulate ourselves for another successful triumph. In this inventory, you'll break down your week and figure out your successes and failures (which aren't really failures—I like to call them "research insights") so that you can integrate every bit of knowledge you picked up.

After you've done seven nights of your daily inventory, set aside some time to do the weekly check-in. Take a moment and look at your nightly inventory from the week. (This shouldn't take long if you keep them short.)

Once you've read them, come back and answer the questions for the weekly inventory here:

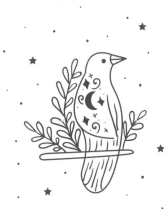

- ★ What are three lessons you learned this week?
- ★ What are three successes you had this week?
- ★ What are three research insights you picked up this week?
- ★ How well have you taken care of yourself?
- ★ How can you take even better care of yourself next week?
- ★ In what ways can you be kinder to yourself next week?

Monthly Inventory

I know this is cliché, but the older I get, the faster the months seem to fly by. A monthly check-in will allow you to develop the clarity you've gotten from the daily and weekly inventories into an even broader perspective. A month is a really good amount of time for us to be able to track our progress, our awareness, and our accountability to ourselves. I don't want you to feel any guilt here, either; we are all just human. We need breaks, and things come up. But if you really want to move the needle on your shadow work, make a commitment to keep coming back to it no matter what.

> ### Consider
>
> How well did you take care of yourself this month? How can you take even better care of yourself next month? How can you be kinder to yourself next month?

This one might take a little longer, so set a timer (about thirty minutes or so) to look over your daily and weekly inventories. You don't need to read them word for word, but glance through them and look for any overarching themes or patterns that stick out to you. Sit back, close your eyes for a bit, and remember all the good moments you had over the last thirty days. Take a few

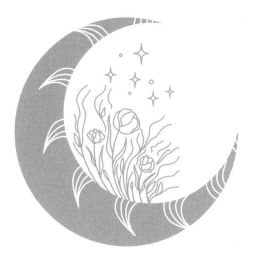

deep breaths and really sink into those lessons from your weekly inventories. When you're ready, answer the following questions:

* ★ What was the overarching theme of the last month?
* ★ What are the three biggest lessons for you to think on?
* ★ What are the three major successes for you to reflect on?
* ★ What are the three relevant research insights for you to process?

Inventory When Triggered

Now that you have some nervous system tools to turn off the stress response, you can manage a trigger without going off the deep end. Good—bravo! Now we have a little gold nugget of info we can take through our inventory and extract the essence of what the trigger is pointing to. First, make sure your stress response is indeed turned off before you go through this inventory, and just be aware you may need your nervous system tools again afterward (don't skip this step) because writing about the trigger may very well trigger you again.

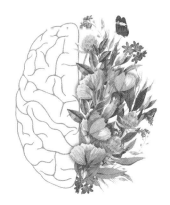

Visualize a Better Outcome

Remember that you are safe, you are secure, you are strong. Triggers do not mean you are doing something wrong. If anything, your willingness to gain more awareness from them means you are doing something right. These questions, and the process of reprogramming your subconscious (by visualizing a better outcome), will dismantle the emotional charge behind the trigger. Afterward, you won't have a strong reaction to this trigger any longer. What I mean is, eventually the trigger will not upset you. It will not trigger you—it will just be a circumstance without any emotion tied to it.

★ What is the trigger scenario? Does this trigger look familiar?

★ List the other times this trigger has shown up for you.

★ Do you have any idea what the trigger is pointing to within you that is unhealed? If so, what is it, and what caused it?

★ If not, continue to leave this question in your conscious awareness.

★ Write down any insights that come to mind.

★ What is a better outcome that you would like to reprogram the trigger with?

★ Reprogram at least ten times. Come back and write about how you feel afterward. Has the emotional reaction to the trigger subsided?

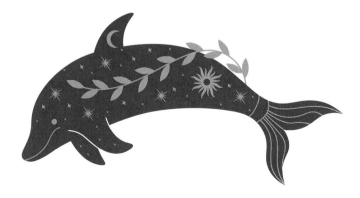

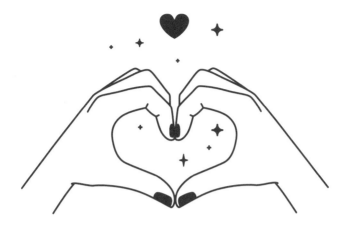

Inventory When Resentful or Envious

When I think of resentment, I think of a quote that describes it as "drinking poison hoping the other person will drop dead." In other words, you are the one poisoning yourself with negative thoughts and beliefs. They might be how you feel about yourself deep down, or they might be how you feel about behaviors and traits you were never allowed to express. You might be surprised, but envy also comes from the same place. These are both tools used by the shadow to remain hidden from your awareness. With envy, however, you're projecting your golden shadow, and you are triggered due to feeling unable to embody that which you witness in the other person.

Looking Closer

Don't let resentment fester inside of you because it's toxic energy. Envy holds some powerful embodiment magic; you just need to turn your attention inward instead of outward and lean into that which sparks envy within you. Now you have this potent tool to help you discharge the emotion and discover what it is your shadow is projecting outwardly. You will know from the daily inventory when you are resentful, and you will know when you are envious.

When either one of these emotions arises, come back to this inventory:

* What are the circumstances? What are you feeling?
* In what way does this person's behavior or trait trigger you?
* Do you ever exhibit this behavior or trait? When you do, how is it different from the person you are projecting onto? (It probably isn't, if you think about it.)
* Can you find some kindness for them since you also do the same thing sometimes?
* If you don't do the same thing, why don't you ever exhibit this trait or behavior?
* Who told you not to behave this way? What would happen if you allowed yourself to behave this way sometimes? Would there be any benefit?

Inventory When Feeling Disconnected

When you feel disconnected, it can be very triggering, especially when you feel like you are not included in the "tribe." The reason for this is the way the nervous system is wired for connection. To our ancestors, it was very important to make sure we belonged to the community. If we did not, we could starve, or be at the mercy of predators of all shapes and sizes. If there was someone in our

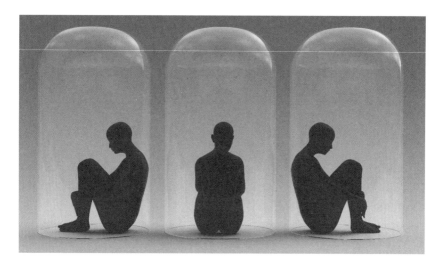

village who hated us and wanted to see us kicked out, that could potentially be a death sentence. We have a myriad of reasons to feel disconnected in this digital age. Less and less do we turn to the ones right next to us for conversation and reciprocity. Instead, we look at glowing screens and seek out some kind of connection and meaning to our existence there.

Disconnection is extremely uncomfortable; it makes many people feel depressed and completely lethargic. Your stress response turns on, and then it needs time to come back to equilibrium. Feeling disconnected for no valid reason has less to do with outside circumstances than you might think: It stems from your thoughts and trauma. Unpack what's making you feel disconnected. This way you'll have a practical tool to turn to when you need it.

- ★ What, if any, are the circumstances causing you to feel disconnected?
- ★ What thoughts are running through your head when you feel like this?
- ★ What thoughts preceded this feeling? Really take time to figure this out.
- ★ Is there any evidence that you should feel disconnected right now?
- ★ Has anyone actually disconnected or excluded you from anything?

If you have a valid reason to feel disconnected, allow yourself to feel the grief that comes up for you. Don't try to push it away or change it. Just allow it, and you'll be surprised how quickly it passes. If you do not have valid evidence as to why you should feel disconnected, then I want you to go and look for evidence to prove to your brain that this isn't true. Write down all the people you are connected to and how. Look at the list again and again, proving to yourself that you are in fact connected to others.

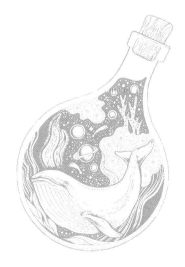

Your brain will want to bring up thoughts over and over that try to prove you should feel disconnected. That's just the way our minds have evolved. Just say, "Thank you, brain. I know. I am safe. It's okay."

Essential Journaling Prompts

Use these essential journaling prompts that you worked on throughout this book in your own journal to continue your shadow work. Revisit and revise your answers often to get a sense of your growth and progress.

★ Did you encounter any examples of golden shadow that offered a creative spark or integration of a repressed talent or gift? If so, how will you commit to embodying this talent or gift in the future?

★ Do you have a close friend that you feel is like your sibling? Write about your relationship and how you interact. What do you think is the benefit of having a person to foster opposition in such close proximity to you?

★ Has your shadow ever revealed itself with this friend? Can you see your shadow in this friend? Do they do things that you judge harshly? Do they aggravate you in certain ways? Do you disagree or fight about anything?

★ List the five most impactful times you ever felt rejected. How did these moments mold you into a false version of yourself? What did you internalize from these moments of rejection? In what ways are you still protecting yourself from being rejected in the same way?

★ What are you actively suppressing that you don't consciously know about? If you stopped suppressing some of the items on your list, what would embodying them look and feel like?

★ Write about a moment where you felt really connected to the source (the universe, God, nature, family, or yourself). Now, write about a moment where you felt really disconnected and lost. What did these moments teach you?

★ Who in your life would you label as good? Who would you label as bad? Take your lists and switch them. How are the good also bad and the bad also good? Lean into this new viewpoint.

★ Are there any emotions you have been avoiding lately? When do you know you are using coping mechanisms to avoid feeling something?

★ How can you applaud your own victories more often? How can you show up feeling like a hero every day?

★ Make a list of the times in your past when you feel like your inner child suffered. If you were a small child (around one to seven years old), how would you take care of yourself if you were sad? Make a list of how you would talk to yourself and treat yourself with love and kindness.

★ What does your inner child need most from you? Take a moment to pause and ask them. Make a list in order of priority. Set aside ten to fifteen minutes each day to give your inner child something from the list.

★ What are your five most impactful traumatic memories? What did you feel in your body during each of these moments? What is the core feeling left behind from each of the previous memories?

★ What are the three biggest triggers you can remember? What did they make you feel like, and what was the result? What is the shadow trying to show you through another person?

★ What feelings is your shadow asking you to lean into? What steps can you take to lean into these feelings?

★ Do you know what the triggers are pointing to within you that is unhealed? If so, what is it, and what caused it?

★ If you feel disconnected from others, allow yourself to feel the grief that comes up for you. Don't try to push it away or change it. Just allow it, and you'll be surprised how quickly it passes. If you do not have valid evidence as to why you should feel disconnected, then I want you to go and look for evidence to prove to your brain that this isn't true. Write down all the people you are connected to and how. Look at the list again and again, proving to yourself that you are in fact connected to others.

❋ ❋ ❋

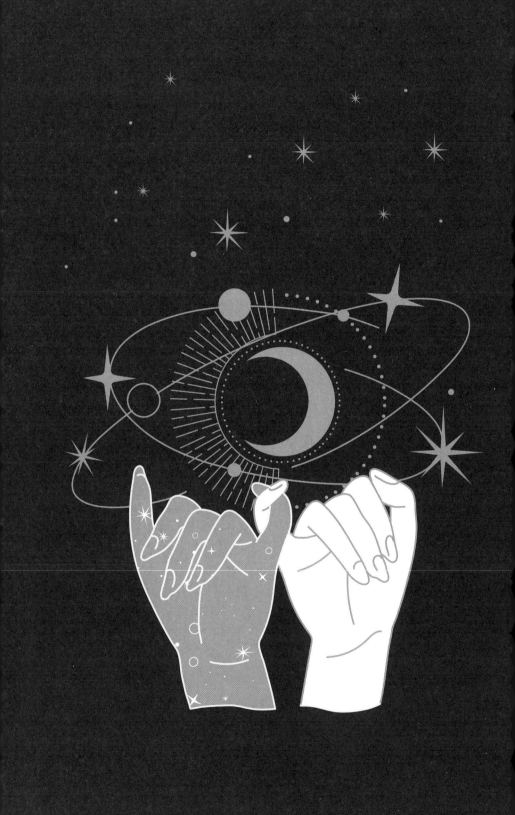

CONCLUSION

Now you can see that your shadow is an integral part of your psyche. You have learned how it helps to guide you along your hero's journey by revealing where you still need more healing. You learned new perspectives by asking yourself the difficult questions that provoked an uncovering of your deepest truths. In doing so, you learned what lines you cross against your true nature to keep up the appearances of your ego. Now the work lies in remembering how to remain a clear channel for your higher self: a powerful, unapologetic version of who you are fundamentally, without repressing and hiding any portions of yourself.

I believe throughout the course of this book you have gained a brand-new sense of your *dark sidekick*, also known as the shadow. You have caught glimpses and perhaps even discovered and developed a truly identifiable sense of this portion of you. This is my invitation for you: take it further and continue on this journey of shadow discovery. This book was not meant to be a casual one-off meeting of the shadow, but rather the start of a deep connection with these lost parts of yourself. That is the main reason I have dedicated a whole chapter to supplying you with inventories. I believe these will help you gain a sense of clarity both in your daily life and in times when you feel troubled by something that's happened. As you progress, it will get easier to see your shadow in plain sight. After the short time we've worked together, you have been sharpening your skills and learning how to spot its presence. You now understand how all strong feelings that come to the surface for you (unless you are suddenly the victim of unprecedented trauma) are simply emotions bubbling up that indeed already existed within you. Projection will become more and more apparent until the point where you will be able to catch yourself before the judgment even slips out of your mouth.

Envy and resentment will begin to spark inquiry within you instead of shameful emotions. You have learned to turn inward and foster a new appreciation for the ways your shadow signals to you when something feels out of alignment within. Let us always remember the shadow uses the only tools it possesses to gain your attention—and since triggers will accomplish that immediately, they are used readily. Our repressed self is always seeking healing. Your comfort comes secondary to the desire for the integrated self to be realized. It's hard to react to a trigger as intensely as you once did, now that you know there is a little gold nugget of your authentic self waiting to be discovered and embodied underneath it. Sure, we will always have emotions and emotional reactions, but when you are deeply aware of exactly where they are stemming from, it becomes easier and easier to treat yourself with the utmost kindness and unconditional self-love. Each day I work with the shadow and its concepts, I am truly amazed that our intelligent design includes a perfect internal self-discovery system set up to consistently guide us to heal childhood wounds and traumatic incidents. The shadow repeats the cycle because it craves integration. The subconscious mind feels comfortable because the situation is familiar. And the nervous system is frazzled, running on overdrive because of the constant triggers and stimulation.

I hope this book has made you keenly aware of how your shadow will guide you toward situations where healing of your core wounds is possible. In the same vein, I want you to understand that you actually have the power to change your knee-jerk reactions and unconscious behaviors that perpetuate exactly what you consciously think you *do not* want. When we run around avoiding emotions, the cycle is endless. Leaning into uncomfortable emotions is a prerequisite for reaching higher levels of consciousness. The more you create space to lean into discomfort, inevitably more space will open up for you to experience joy, happiness, and authentic connection with your loved ones. Take the time to really know yourself in an intimate way. Question everything, then make time to question everything all over again, including the conclusions you have already realized. Self-actualization is a lifelong process of unraveling your own mind and the inner workings that have been set in place by your predecessors and the unconscious desire we all have to belong. The only way to truly know oneself is to know all of the unconscious and repressed parts too—for, as you've witnessed, they are indeed the true guiding principle of consciousness. If we do not take the time to discover ourselves here, self-realization is not possible.

✳   ✳   ✳

REFERENCES AND RESOURCES

Books

Bane, Rosanne. *Dancing in the Dragon's Den: Rekindling the Creative Fire in Your Shadow.* York Beach, ME: Nicolas-Hays, 1999.

Nagoski, Emily, and Amelia Nagoski. *Burnout: The Secret to Unlocking the Stress Cycle* New York: Ballantine Books, 2020.

Rosenberg, Stanley. *Accessing the Healing Power of the Vagus Nerve: Self-Help Exercises for Anxiety, Depression, Trauma, and Autism.* Berkeley, CA: North Atlantic Books, 2017.

van der Kolk, Bessel. *The Body Keeps the Score: Brain, Mind, and Body in the Healing of Trauma.* New York: Viking Press, 2014.

Walker, Pete. *Complex PTSD: From Surviving to Thriving.* Lafayette, CA: Azure Coyote Publishing, 2013.

Wodehouse, P.G. *Uneasy Money.* New York: D. Appleton & Company, 1916.

Zweig, Connie and Jeremiah Abrams, eds. *Meeting the Shadow: The Hidden Power of the Dark Side of Human Nature.* New York: TarcherPerigee, 1991.

Web Pages

Aybar, Susan. "4 Somatic Therapy Exercises for Healing from Trauma" https://psychcentral.com/lib/somatic-therapy-exercises-for-trauma.

Brown, Kelly. "What Is Step 10 of AA?" https://alcoholrehabhelp.org/treatment/alcoholics-anonymous/step-10/.

Earl, Ronnie. "Step 10: Daily Inventory" https://sobrietyfreedom.com/step-10-daily-inventory/.

Hayes, Kacey. "What Is Emotional Buffering, and Why Do HSPs Do It?" https://highlysensitiverefuge.com/what-is-emotional-buffering-and-why-do-hsps-do-it/.

Hoshaw, Crystal. "6 Ways to Give Your Nervous System a Break" https://www.cmbody-ayurveda.com/blog/ways-to-give-your-nervous-system-a-break.

Innis, Jeri. "Calming a Wigged Out Autonomic Nervous System Using the Vagus Nerve" https://www.innisintegrativetherapy.com/blog/2017/11/21/calming-a-wigged-out-autonomic-nervous-system-using-the-vagus-nerve.

Jeffrey, Scott. "Psychological Projection: Reclaim the Best in You" https://scottjeffrey.com/psychological-projection/.

Matson, Marquis. "Top 10 Best Restorative Yoga Poses That Even Your Grandmother Could Do" https://bookretreats.com/blog/restorative-yoga-poses/.

Puusa, Seppo. "3-2-1 Technique" https://www.acneeinstein.com/cfl/3-2-1-technique/.

Seol, Simone. "145. The surprising reason you're not booking clients" https://www.simonegraceseol.com/podcast/not-booking-clients.

Sinha Clinic. "What Are Brain Waves?" https://www.sinhaclinic.com/what-are-brainwaves/.

Spayde, Jon. "How to Stop Projecting" https://experiencelife.lifetime.life/article/how-to-stop-projecting/.

Stoddart, Tim. "5 Daily Inventory Questions That Will Keep You Sober" https://sobernation.com/daily-inventory/.

Windle, Nicole. "10 Restorative Yoga Poses to Chill Out Right Now" https://www.brettlarkin.com/restorative-yoga-poses/.

IMAGE CREDITS

ABOUT THE AUTHOR

Stephanie Kirby is a devout student of energy medicine, having studied across various subject fields and utilized practical applications of healing tools and practices on herself. She is a twice-certified hatha and kundalini yoga instructor, herbalist, occultist, and expert on the inner workings of the mind and the symbolism it uses. Stephanie traveled to many different countries in search of answers. In 2013, she studied Buddhism, meditation, and yoga as a path to enlightenment, learning from wise sages in Dharamsala, India. Her life's work has been to study people and the process of integrating and profoundly healing on a soul level. She believes our true purpose in life is to discover the pathway back to a whole self, which is only made possible by confronting one's shadow.

With shadow work, Stephanie finally felt like she was understood after she learned to understand herself—and the origins of her negative thinking patterns and destructive coping mechanisms. Suddenly, her abusive self-talk had a context that could be pinpointed and narrowed down, observed, and then destroyed. The cruel voices in her head could be identified and named after their originators. After years of self-discovery, she realized the chronic illness symptoms she suffered for over seven years could be traced back to repetitive thoughts of feeling unwell and constant tensed muscles attempting to armor her body from danger. All the while, her stress response ran rampant. She was simultaneously expecting and modeling these sensations of discomfort because her nervous system was blown out from running on overdrive since childhood. The process of deconditioning the mind is unique and to be discovered by each individual as the process unfolds with the shadow's steady guidance. This book serves as Stephanie's unique point of view as to how to undertake this process. The "Consider" questions, "Take Action" boxes, journaling prompts, and activities are specific to her approach and offer many insights to work with.

INDEX

A

abuse
  childhood development and, 61
  complex PTSD (CPTSD), 75
  coping mechanisms for, 99
  familiarity of, 24
  Fawn response, 82
  nervous system response, 74
  ongoing threat of, 30
  patterns of, 24, 30
  trauma from, 30, 98
  therapy for, 52
adrenaline, 88
alpha brain waves, 45
amygdala, 74, 88, 93, 94
ancestors
  ancestral trauma, 40, 41
  hero's journey and, 35
  influence of, 35
  knowledge from, 40
  struggles of, 40
  trauma and, 35
authenticity
  acceptance of, 18–19
  approval vs., 27
  rejection and, 23

B

beta brain waves, 45, 46
Bilateral Stimulation, 93
The Body Keeps the Score (Bessel van
  der Kolk), 72, 91–92
box breathing, 87
brain. *See also* nervous system
  alpha waves, 45
  amygdala, 74, 88, 93, 94
  beta waves, 45, 46
  delta waves, 46, 93
  evolution of, 86
  frontal lobe, 45
  gamma waves, 45
  hippocampus, 74
  hypothalamus, 74, 88
  limbic system, 74, 87, 94
  mirror neurons, 63
  myelin, 89
  neurons, 45, 63
  pain response, 47
  prefrontal cortex, 74
  theta waves, 46

C

childhood. *See also* inner child
  abuse in, 61, 82, 98
  adults behaving as, 33
  ancestral trauma in, 41
  approval in, 27
  caregivers and, 27
  complex PTSD (CPTSD), 75
  curiosity in, 61, 64
  disconnection in, 60
  emotional memories, 76
  environmental dynamics, 31, 63
  familiar patterns in, 31
  influence of, 59, 68
  internalization in, 59, 62
  lack of empowerment in, 68
  mirror neurons, 63
  observation in, 61
  parents and, 19, 21
  pressures, 65–66
  programming in, 19, 21, 57,
    60–61
  regression to, 33
  shadow creation in, 60
  stability in, 59, 61
  trauma, 13, 41, 52, 61–62, 64,
    67, 68, 82, 90, 98
  trust and, 59
Child's Pose (Bālāsana), 81
cinema, 14–15
complex PTSD (CPTSD), 75, 77
confirmation bias, 51
conscious mind, 8, 45
cortisol, 82, 88

D

daily inventory, 107, 108–109, 113
delta brain waves, 46, 93
disconnection, 114–115, 117
Disowned Self, 28–29

E

ego
  definition of, 11
  development of, 12, 61, 63
  discomfort and, 19
  Disowned Self and, 28–29
  function of, 11, 14
  influence of, 19
  Lost Self and, 29
  necessity of, 17
  parenthood and, 61
  projection and, 100
  shadow and, 7, 8, 11–12, 14

  storytelling and, 25
  suppression and, 28
envy, 13, 14, 100, 113

F

False Self, 27, 28, 29
Fawn response, 74, 82, 90
Fight response, 74, 82, 86, 90, 93
Fish Pose (Matsyasana), 77
Flight response, 74, 82, 86, 90, 93
four-F response, 74, 82, 86, 87, 90,
  93, 94
Freeze response, 74, 82, 90
Freud, Sigmund, 7
frontal lobe, 45

G

gamma brain waves, 45
golden shadow
  beneficial aspects of, 13–14
  definition of, 13
  envy and, 13–14, 100, 113
  repressed talent and, 14, 116

H

hero's journey
  ancestors and, 35, 40
  definition of, 35, 39
  hero development, 38
  scapegoats, 42
  ubiquity of, 39–40
  visualization and, 38, 42
hippocampus, 74
hypothalamus, 74, 88

I

individuation, 8, 68–69
inner child. *See also* childhood
  compassion for, 66
  complex PTSD (CPTSD), 75
  conformity and, 64
  connecting to, 62
  empowerment of, 67–69
  grieving for, 62
  healing, 59, 66
  influence of, 59
  internalization and, 59
  journal prompts, 117
  nervous system and, 59
  parental influence on, 60–61
  playtime for, 69
  trauma and, 59–60, 64–65, 67
inventory
  daily inventory, 107, 108–109,
    113